DIABETES NUTRITION
and
ELECTRIC MEDICINE

SAM RAMBI M.D.

ISBN-13: 978-1543111125

ISBN-10: 1543111122

Dedicated
to
Ziggy
The light of my life

CONTENTS

RIBOSE 5-CARBON SUGAR

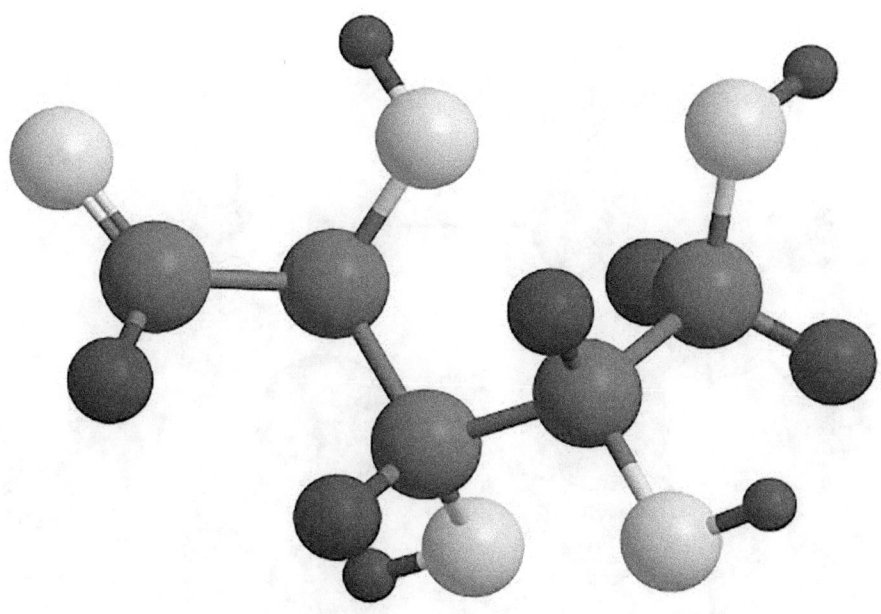

GLUCOSE 6-CARBON SUGAR

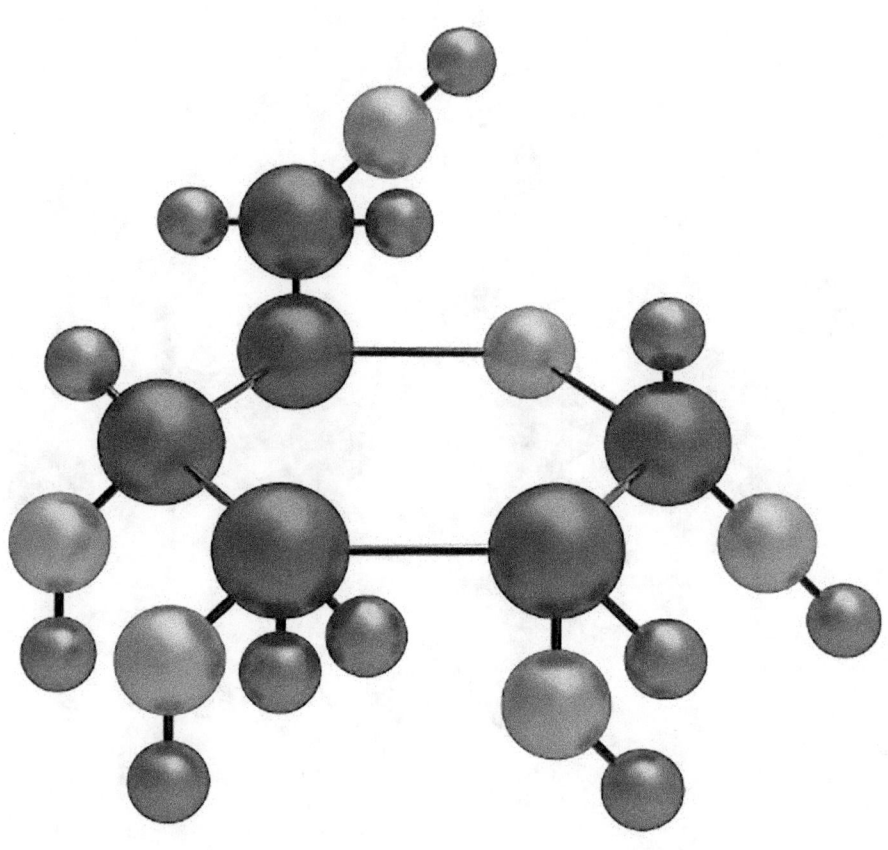

OXYGEN

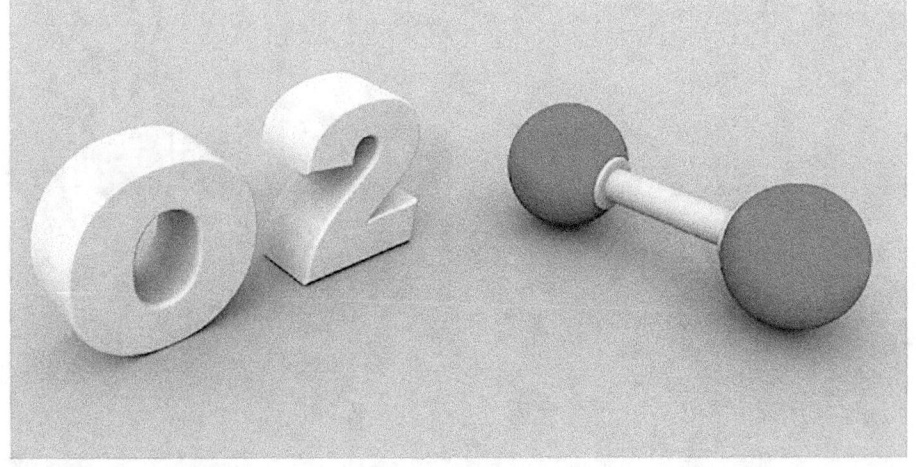

ATP

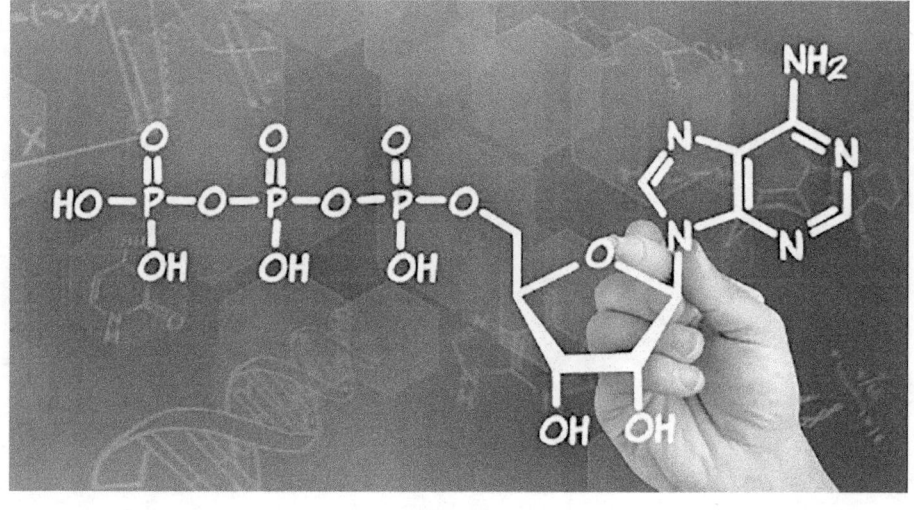

MITOCHONDRIAL FUNCTION

1. ATP synthesis.
2. Synthesis own organic substances.
3. Education own ribosomes.

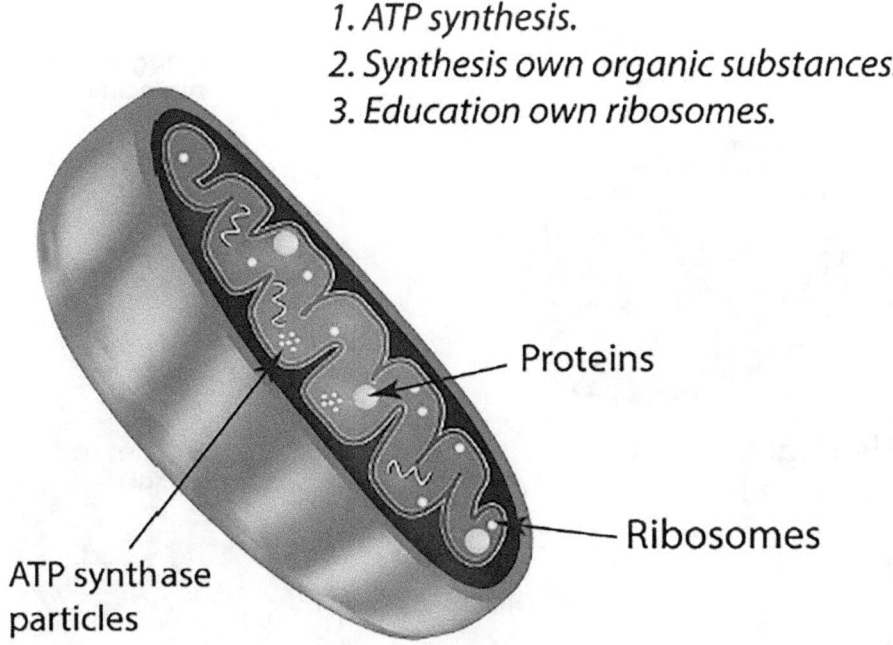

Proteins

Ribosomes

ATP synthase particles

HUMAN HEMOGLOBIN

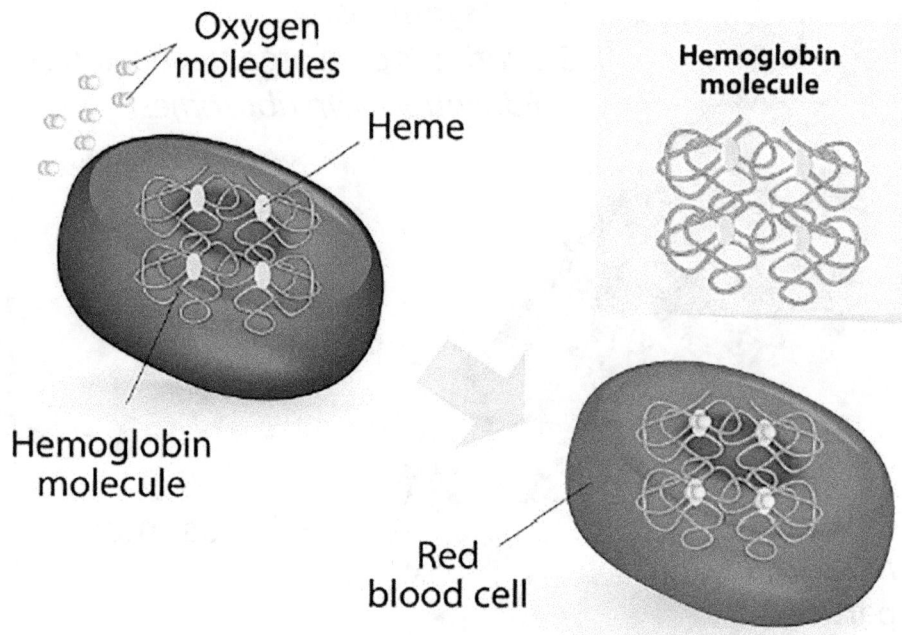

Oxygen molecules

Heme

Hemoglobin molecule

Hemoglobin molecule

Red blood cell

HUMAN INSULIN

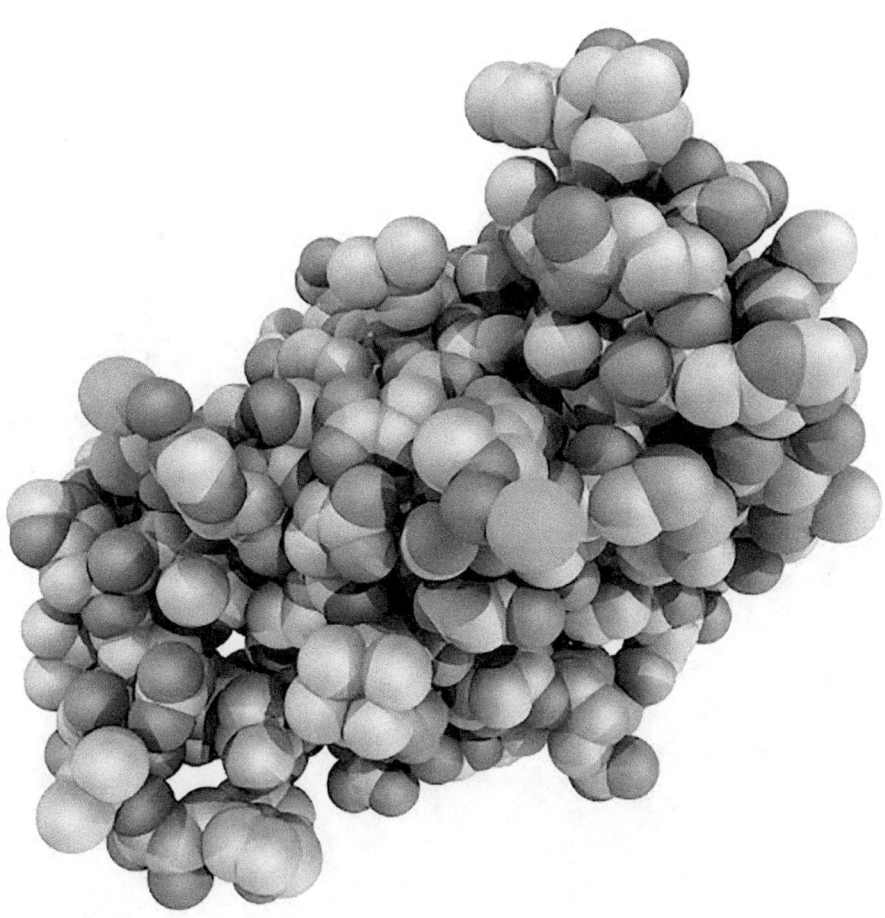

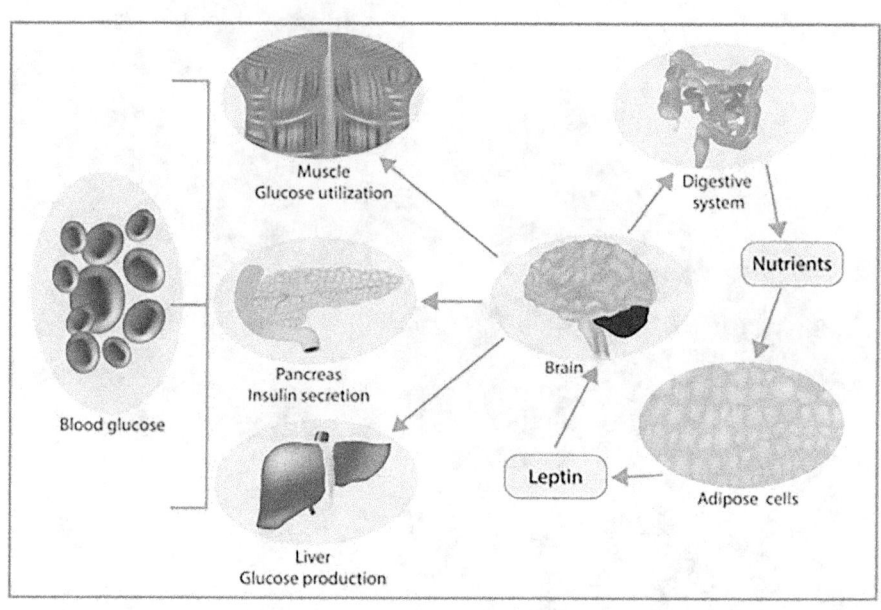

Muscle
Glucose utilization

Digestive
system

Nutrients

Pancreas
Insulin secretion

Brain

Blood glucose

Leptin

Adipose cells

Liver
Glucose production

FOREWORD

Every effort has been made to keep this document free of excessive verbiage. It is intended to make reading it as easy as possible, and not waste your time by padding with extra wording that does not advance the narrative.

I hope to stick to the facts as closely as possible.

Information on diabetes is scattered far and wide in the medical literature, and an attempt has been made to draw information together in a meaningful way.

This monograph is a specific denial of giving medical advice. Under no circumstances is this monograph advice on what you should do personally in seeking medical care. Always depend on your personal physician for advice and management.

A whole diabetes industry has been built up. For the most part, treatment has been directed at managing diabetes, not curing it. Many programs are offered and claim to get rid of your dependency on drugs, and reestablish your natural sensitivity to insulin. Some of these programs depend on fasting and green juices to reestablish insulin sensitivity.

Fasting resets insulin sensitivity.

There is a prediction that a massive increase of the diabetic population is about to occur. It is unlikely that the human genome has changed rapidly enough to be the genetic basis for the surge in diabetic numbers. Our genetic evolution environment does not match our current environment and diet. What passes for familial diabetes is more likely social. Families tend to have similar lifestyles and dietary habits.

There is also a prediction that Type 3 diabetes is on the increase... also known as Alzheimer's disease. The financial burdens for taking care of predicted volume of Alzheimer's patients threatens to bankrupt the nation.

A definite linkage is/may soon be solved since there is some commonalty between diabetes and Alzheimer's disease. The McGovern School of Medicine in Houston Texas is investigating a molecular connection between the biology of diabetes and Alzheimer's.

A misfolded protein molecule is present in brain tissue of AZ patients and a similar misfolded protein is found in the islet of Langerhans cells in the pancreas which produces insulin. Beta amyloid and abnormal amylin clusters are found in the brain of AZ patients. Insulin is necessary for establishing memory, learning and thought processes. Amyloid is believed to destroy normal brain cells and their connections.

The misfolded protein destroys insulin function in the pancreas. The insulin which is formed, is abnormal, so it piles up in circulation, resulting in higher measured circulating insulin, but not sensitive enough to produce normal glucose metabolism. 75% of diabetics are likely to develop Alzheimer's disease (type 3 diabetes). It is easy to see how diabetes and AZ may be associated if this research is confirmed.

If the answer to diabetes is solved, perhaps the solution to Alzheimer's disease can be found.

Dr. Dale E. Bredersen has a new explanation of Alzheimer's Disease. He outlines beta amyloid as a process whereby the brain makes amyloid as a protective mechanism against factors which are attacking normal function of the brain. He has developed a protocol called DeCODE and claims to have essentially reversed Alzheimer's Disease. He defines three types of AZ and postulates that inflammation, dietary deficiencies and toxins are the major insults to the brain. They are reversible to a large degree, especially if the correct diagnosis is made and vigorously treated.

The ApoE4 gene is critically important but nobody should die of AZ if he is right. ApoE4 is a fat carrier molecule.

There is a good chance that exposure to toxins and chemicals in recent years has a lot to do with the rise of diabetes. We still don't know if the effect of genetically modified foods has anything to do with the rise of diabetes and a strenuous effort is being made to prevent us from getting good scientific information. A simple thing like having a label to identify products as GMO or not GMO has become a big problem. Some parties are strongly resisting the labelling of foods with GMO contents. We have a revolving door in which politicians become regulators and lobbyists.

So the lines are becoming blurred.

Uninformed politicians are influenced by lobbyists who are more often than not looking out for big business rather than consumers.

Screening for diabetes is likely to discover pre-diabetic status, and permit preventative regimens to be executed sooner rather than later. The search for stem cells to restore insulin production and sensitivity might provide a solution. Hopefully current investigations will open new doors in managing and treating diabetes.

Any errors of fact in this book are the sole fault and responsibility of the author. I invite you to go along on the journey with me.

BEGINNINGS

Today started like just another routine day in your life. You didn't have a care in the world. Later you were dropping by your doctor's office to get some results for blood tests that were drawn at a previous routine visit.

Your Dr. was very serious as he greeted you. These results show that you are a diabetic.

In an instant your life was changed forever. How did he decide? Your hemoglobin A1c is up, and your fasting glucose is elevated too. Maybe he will order a glucose tolerance test with insulin each time your blood is drawn, but maybe not. The A1c is sufficient to follow your progress. There are tables that show what glucose ranges represent matching levels of matching A1c.

HEMOGLOBIN A1c

But what is A1c and why is it important?

When you were in your mother's uterus, your hemoglobin was slightly different from that in your mother's circulation. Hers was adult hemoglobin and yours was fetal hemoglobin.

After the miracle of birth, your hemoglobin converted to adult hemoglobin too. But a tiny fraction of fetal hemoglobin persists in your red cell membrane.

Roughly fifty years ago, measuring fetal hemoglobin was done by dissolving red cells and applying the solution to a paper substrate. It was connected to an electrical current and allowed to run for a fixed period of time.

Proteins with similar weights and similar electric charge migrated together in bands on the paper substrate. Biological stains permitted visual identification of the different hemoglobin proteins. Now you can see the separate fractions. These bands were cut apart and eluted. Colored liquid elution could now be measured for concentrations of fetal hemoglobin.

The bands were assigned names. Band A had finer separations. Sub group A had numbers and letters for identification. Hemoglobin A1c was part of band A, line1, subsection "c". Shortened version nomenclature is Hb A1c!!!

That is reported as a test result today.

A WORD OF CAUTION

Individuals who have sickle-cell trait or people with thalassemia disease and sickle cell anemia have abnormal red cells with variation of the usual 90 day life. Their red cell population is less than 90 days but nobody knows how long they remain in circulation. So there is less saturation of A1c. As a result they could have a lower A1c together with a higher circulating plasma glucose. Their physicians need to take this discrepancy into consideration when managing their diabetes.

Why is A1c important for diabetics?

Because somebody discovered that the persistent fetal hemoglobin has an affinity for circulating glucose in your plasma. The higher the concentration of freely circulating glucose, the larger the amount of glucose that becomes fixed to the fetal hemoglobin of the red cells.

Primary function of hemoglobin in your red cell is to loosely grab oxygen from your pulmonary microcirculation and exchange it for carbon dioxide dissolved in the interstitial fluid surrounding the cells that make up your tissue.

The hemoglobin in your red cells in circulation has a greater concentration of oxygen than in interstitial fluid of your tissues. Oxygen diffuses across the intervening cell membranes and is eventually taken up by the mitochondria to enter the Krebs Cycle for producing ATP.

Oxygen is grabbed loosely by the hemoglobin and is released by a catalase reaction. At the center of the hemoglobin molecule is the mineral iron. You need enough iron to carry the oxygen along. Not enough iron and you get iron deficiency anemia. Too much iron and you get hemochromatosis that results in bronze diabetes. This is a genetic disorder. The gene resides on the short arm of chromosome 6. The gene is relatively common, but disease is only expressed as a recessive trait disorder so you need two copies of the gene to get the disease.

Those with the disease absorb too much iron from the gut. Excess iron is deposited in the skin, heart, lungs, liver, gut and brain. It could result in skin discoloration, (gray or bronze skin) heart failure, diabetes, liver cancer, pulmonary hemosiderosis, cancer in the colon (red meat is high in iron, hence the advice to avoid eating too much red meat).

Iron deposits in the brain causes degenerative brain conditions as Parkinson's and Alzheimer's.

Cure for excess iron is removal of blood. The removed blood must be discarded. It is not fit for transfusion.

Once upon a time, bloodletting was practiced to cure "whatever ailed you". One of our former presidents reportedly died of overly aggressive blood-letting.

Menstruating females have some degree of protection up to menopause. Beyond that point they lose their advantage over males with respect to heart disease. Their regular loss of blood and overall lifetime lower iron level, is thought to be the reason why females outlive males. A blood test for ferritin allows you to keep track of the iron in circulation.

By the time oxygen has traveled from the lung to mitochondria it has crossed about nine sets of double membranes. Hence the importance of having membranes of good quality essential fatty acids.

On the day when blood was drawn to test for hemoglobin A1c, your red cell population had a mixture of red cells of different ages. New red cells are released from your red bone marrow.

KIDNEYS

Your kidneys produce a protein called erythropoietin which stimulates stem cells in the bone marrow to manufacture new red cells and release them continuously into circulation. The life of a new red blood cell is about ninety days or three months. Circulating blood is a mixture of cells that was released today or at least this week for sure, as well as each and every single day ranging from one day to ninety days.

That is why an A1c test represents an average of your blood glucose over ninety days and you need to repeat A1c tests every ninety days. The oldest ninety day cells are removed from circulation. Senescent red cells are removed from circulation by the spleen.

Hemoglobin A1c charts have been built to give your doctor an idea of how your diabetic control is working.

%A1c	Average Glucose	Range of Glucoset
5	97	76–120
6	126	100–152
7	154	123–185
8	183	147–217
9	212	170–249
10	240	193–282
11	269	217–314
12	298	240–347
13	326	260–380
14	355	290–410
15	384	310–440
16	413	330–480
17	441	460–510
18	470	480–540
19	499	510–570

As your out-of-control diabetes becomes more severe, your glucose rises and falls within a higher range on a daily basis. Percentage tables are available to make it easier for your doctor. He/she can figure your glucose average levels over the previous 90 days. It takes the guess work out of deciding how all your lifestyle or diet, nutrition, medication, exercises etc. is reflected in your diabetic control.

If you are diagnosed with diabetes you will have to make life style changes. A big hurdle is first of all to accept that you have diabetes. That acceptance may be slow in coming, but you will eventually adjust mentally. You then are ready to do what you need to do in order to live an orderly life.

COMPLICATIONS OF DIABETES

Uncontrolled diabetes is very unforgiving. The complications are dire. Every part of your body is vulnerable. High levels of circulating glucose is toxic to the endothelial cells of your blood vessels. In the eye, blood vessels leak, resulting in diabetic retinopathy. So you'll need to be examined by your opthalmologist regularly.

Diabetics develop heart disease slowly but surely. And diabetes is a multi - system problem. It affects your heart, eyes, kidneys, nerves, gastrointestinal tract and liver. Diabetes affects your entire body.

Your kidneys go bad. Diabetes is the most frequent reason for kidney transplants. The amount of glucose in circulation overwhelms the ability of the renal loops of Henle to reabsorb glucose and electrolytes as they stream by in the blood vessels of the glomerulus. It is as if you are counting individual cars as they drive by. You lose count if the stream of traffic becomes faster than you can count.

Eventually glucose begins to spill over into your urine. The higher the glucose, the greater the spill.

You'll have to urinate more often. In olden times, you might taste the glucose in a urine specimen, hence the term "sugar diabetes". Nowadays you dip a test strip to analyze the degree of glycosuria.

You lose sleep because you need to get up more often to empty your bladder. The specific gravity of your urine increases as the glycosuria increases. The basement membrane in your kidneys become leaky, and you'll get proteins spilling into the urine that is excreted.

Your doctor uses protein tests to measure how much protein you are losing, which is an indication of the severity of your renal disease. As you lose proteins, you develop edema because there is insufficient osmolar attraction to keep water inside your vasculature.

You are born with a fixed number of glomeruli during nephrogenesis while developing within your mother's uterus. At birth you have all the glomeruli that you will ever have. At this time, it is believed that you cannot grow new glomeruli. At one time we believed that new brain cells could not develop. Maybe we will modify our idea about renal cells too some day.

Over your lifetime, you will gradually lose some number of functioning glomeruli. These functioning glomeruli are responsible for filtering out waste and electrolytes and other minerals etc. The Loops of Henle is where active filtration takes place. Some things are filtered out, other things are exchanged actively, and other things are lost without being recovered or exchanged.

Normally, the kidneys are very efficient at keeping circulating proteins inside your vascular system. Inefficient renal function is also measured by the electrolytes that may get flushed out. The kidney loses its ability to govern your internal environment. Renal failure eventually sets in.

The kidneys usually excrete waste products of protein metabolism. You measure BUN (blood urea nitrogen) and creatinine to keep track of kidney function on a continuous basis. Normal kidneys keep these two values low. Failing kidneys do not keep them in normal range. BUN and creatinine gradually increase as renal function decreases.

The amount of blood that can be processed becomes less and less. This is a measure your glomerular filtration rate. Rising urea nitrogen and rising creatinine levels reflect filtration rates heading in the wrong direction. Eventually you will be joining the long list of people who are waiting for a renal transplant.

As a part of normal functioning, kidneys produce renin that regulates blood pressure. Another hormone is calcitrol. It is the active form of Vitamin D and it regulates calcium metabolism. One more function is the production of erythropoietin. It governs the making of new red cells in the bone marrow.

So the kidneys have excretory functions as well as hormonal functions. Two kidneys are better than one but you can survive nicely with one kidney that is working well. That is where living kidney donors come in. While you wait for a compatible donor, renal dialysis is an expensive and time consuming process. As well as an emotionally draining process, it takes control of your life.

Hope is on the way. Dr. Shuvo Roy (UCSF), Dr. William Fussell (Vanderbilt Univ) and Dr. David Hume (Univ of Michigan) have pooled their talents and assembled a bioartificial compact kidney that is implantable into a patient.

It treats end-stage renal disease (ESRD). It replaces external machine dialysis which has become a $30. billion dollar industry. Current funding comes from

NIH and FDA. Stage 2 clinical trials are due to start shortly.

The assembly includes silicon filters capable of 7 nanometer filtration. Human cells from kidney nephrons are part of the filtration which performs many of the biological functions of a native kidney. The filter keeps out immune cells so there is no rejection which is a problem with donor kidneys. This bioartificial kidney could do away with the need for human donors. Be patient. It could be operational in your lifetime.

GUT & GASTROINTESTINAL & NUTRITION

Whatever nutrients get in the bloodstream must be first ingested and then digested and absorbed by crossing the lining membranes of the gut wall. A normal healthy gut has cells lined up adjacent to one another and they are bound together by a protein named zonulin to form tight junctions. There is a simple test to determine if you have a leaky gut. Take a test dose of a mixture of mannose and lactulose. Now check your urine. Normally the mannose is excreted into the urine. But not lactulose.

If you have lactulose in the urine, you have a leaky gut. Two things will help you to cure a leaky gut. One is fasting and the other is taking beef broth.

If these tight junctions lose their integrity, the gut becomes leaky. A leaky gut allows larger protein molecules to enter the bloodstream where they act as antigens which may permit allergies and immune disorders to develop. Nutrients are normally permitted to cross from the gut into circulation, to be transported to the liver for processing.

In the gut itself, the microbiome of bacteria live. These bacteria act upon whatever food is presented by your diet. The number of genes in the bacteria of your gut far exceeds the number of genes that comprise the human genome. This makes epigenetics an important part of modern medicine. It also accounts for the importance of probiotics to establish a favorable balance of the bacteria in your gut.

The gut bacteria help to digest food but they also make vitamins and other nutrients. Carbohydrates that quickly convert to glucose result in spikes in blood sugar levels.

Glucose in the gut is transferred into tissue cells with the help of insulin which is essentially a fat storage hormone.

Insulin is an old molecule historically from a genetic evolutionary standpoint. Insulin is produced in single-celled yeast organisms. That is how old insulin is in the evolutionary chain.

Early in the history of diabetes, insulin was collected from pig pancreas. The protein molecules stimulated resistant antigenic responses, so pig insulin was discontinued. Today Genentech can produce unlimited amounts of insulin. This insulin is not antigenic in humans, and is relatively safe for treatment of diabetics.

The glycemic index is a measure of how fast carbohydrates produce a rise in the blood glucose level when compared with taking pure glucose. Some complex carbohydrates are broken down less rapidly and cause slower rise in blood glucose level. They are low glycemic carbohydrates.

And then, there are slow starches such as potato starch, green banana starch and plantain starch. These slow carbohydrates are not digested in the small bowel. Instead they don't get digested until they reach the large bowel.

There they are digested by bacteria species of the microbiome that feed upon prebiotics. So you need to include prebiotics as part of your diet. Inulin (different from inSulin) is an excellent prebiotic. Slow starch digestion does not cause insulin spikes. Slow starches are digested into fatty acids and those are readily converted into energy, without producing insulin spikes. You can actually convert some regular starch into slow starch. Boil a white potato or a colored sweet potato. Put it into a refrigerator or freezer overnight or for 24 hours. Next day, remove it, thaw out and reheat. A significant amount of regular starch will have been converted to slow starch. This slow starch will be digested and burned as fat, without insulin spike or glucose spike.

As a side note, while glucose is the primary source of energy for the brain, it will happily use fatty acids (ketones) if presented to it as an energy source.

If you are a believer, a ketogenic diet will help you avoid insulin spikes. More fat intake will lead to ketosis and increase ketones. Ketones feed the brain just as easily as when glucose is supplied to the brain.

Ketosis is not the same as ketogenic acidosis which is a pathologic state. Ketogenic acidosis leads to diabetic coma. Abnormal acidity is present. Recovery needs re-establishment of alkalinity with alkaline fluids. (You are healthy in an alkaline pH status). You may monitor ketogenic indices to keep track of your status. You must compare your glucose level to your ketone values.

Glucose must be in units of nmols. If you do not have a meter calibrated for nmol readings, then convert. Glucose mg X 0.055 = nmol/dl ketones. Normal ketone levels are 7 or 8. They reflect the health of your mitochondria.

The golden rule of your life is to produce energy and warmth. That means nutrition has to be ingested and digested. These products of all digestion must go to where the energy factory is located.

That site is the mitochondria which has it's own double layered wall enclosure and its own separate DNA and RNA. Mitochondria have a DNA structure of 37 nucleotides in a circular arrangement. This is reminiscent of bacteria that were pulled into cells by pinocytosis. Eventually those bacteria established a symbiosis and are our modern day mitochondria.

ATP

Nutrients must go through a process of being introduced into a Krebs cycle which requires oxygen. The process results in ATP formation. Your body uses ATP for all its energy requirements.

Supplements which promote an efficient Krebs cycle may include PQQ, niacinamide - riboside and oxaloacetate.

In the mitochondria your biochemistry uses enzymes, nutrients and oxygen to produce ATP. (adenosine triphosphate). 38 molecules of ATP are produced for each aerobic cycle. Only 4 molecules of ATP are produced per anaerobic cycle. Anaerobic metabolism is older than aerobic metabolism. If for some reason aerobic metabolism is interrupted, the body goes as a fallback alternative to anaerobic states but with far fewer ATP molecules produced. Cancer cells revert back to anaerobic glycolysis.

Fat molecules have 147 electrons available and glucose molecules have 36. The Krebs cycle uses an electron chain transport to create ATP. So fats produce more energy than carbohydrates (sugars and starches). More electrons are available.

Oxygen represents more than 40% of the molecular mass of an ATP molecule. Hence the need for good oxygenation which depends on the integrity of healthy cell walls, which in turn depend on a good supply of essential fatty acids.

ATP is constantly being used up, and needs constant new oxygen to regenerate as ADP becomes recycled into ATP.

You probably have less than a pound of ATP at any single moment, but cycle through your body weight of ATP in a twenty four hour period. e.g. a person weighing 150 lbs. will utilize 150 lbs. of ATP in 24 hours but only have 1 pound of ATP at any instant. It has to be regenerated over and over and over.

You need Omega 3 fatty acids and Omega 6 fatty acids with a proper balance of 3 : 6. Ideally there should be 2 or 3 of sixes to each Omega 3. Best of all would be a 1 : 1 ratio which is extremely difficult to obtain. Flax oil and macadamia nut oil are excellent sources of Omega 3 fats.

Regeneration of ATP production must go on continuously. The process uses ribose sugar which has a 5 carbon structure as opposed to glucose which has a 6 carbon structure.

Oxaloacetate is also needed to replenish NAD+ (Nicotinamide adenine dinucleotide) that is an important step of Krebs metabolism which regenerates ATP from ADP. The Krebs cycle operates with ribose as its sugar. It does not use glucose.

Enzymes work best at a slightly alkaline pH. Every pH value corresponds to a specific electrical voltage potential.

More of that later in the section on electricity and health.

OXYGEN

A good supply of oxygen is critical to an efficiently functioning oxidative metabolism environment. The transfer of oxygen goes from higher concentrations at the beginning of the chain, and ending at mitochondria at the other end of the chain.

Your intake of oxygen is dependent on your breathing air that is clean and as high as possible in its oxygen content. You can learn breathing techniques that would maximize the oxygen that is extracted from the air you breathe. Polluted air is bad for your health.

Mitochondria is where the action is. You inherit all of your mitochondria from your mother. None from your father. There are mitochondria everywhere in your body. The highest concentration of all is found in the ovaries of females. Other areas of high concentration are in the prefrontal cortex of the brain, in the retina of the eyes and in the muscles of the heart.

You can generate increasing number of new mitochondria by taking PQQ supplement (Pyroloquinoline). Pterostilbene works together with PQQ as a stimulator of increased mitochondrial biogenesis. As you grow older, the body makes less and less of new mitochondria.

You begin to lose your energy. Regenerating more mitochondria restores your energy. More new mitochondria is akin to increasing a workforce. You become more productive with new mitochondrial biogenesis. More mitochondria increases longevity.

Exposure to sunlight is good for Vitamin D production. Sunlight also increases the electron energy of mitochondria and therefore increases ATP production.

Direct electric current is produced when DHA is exposed to the photons of sunlight.

Apple cider vinegar is also thought to make mitochondria perform more efficiently.

Many ways are possible for increasing oxygen pressure. You can have oxygen delivered in pressurized chambers as in rescue for divers who have the "bends". Diabetic ulcers can be treated with hyperbaric chambers if they are available.

Check AVAZZIA in last chapter.

You can buy oxygen enclosures where the head is outside the enclosure but the body is enclosed and pressurized oxygen source is connected to the enclosure. Using increased pressure, oxygen is absorbed through your skin.

You may have ozone insufflated by rectal catheter.

Oxygen concentrators can extract more oxygen from atmospheric air and taken in through breathing masks such as the practice of exercise with oxygen. (EWOT).

The poor man's way of increasing oxygen is to obtain 35 % food-grade hydrogen peroxide and adding it to chlorine-free water. Start with a few drops and gradually increase on a daily schedule. Adjust the drops of peroxide to taste tolerance. If the taste is unacceptable, reduce the number of drops.

You can buy whole house ozone generators to flood your house with ozone and experience "ocean breeze" inside your house.

Chlorine dioxide has two oxygens available. It carries a negative electrical charge and alkaline pH. Chlorine dioxide is capable of destroying any positively charged molecule. This includes viruses and bacteria, Even drug-resistant MRSA. (Methicillin Resistant Staph Aureus).

Ozone has three oxygen molecules. Food grade peroxide has two oxygens. Chlorine dioxide has two oxygens and water has one oxygen.

You can choose which of them is available to you for immediate use. A medical doctor Dr. Robert Rowen in northern California (Santa Rosa) is the most famous proponent of ozone therapy. He has an ozone therapy practice and teaches other medical providers with hands-on instruction. He is an international expert on ozone and oxygen therapy. He took a team to Africa to treat ebola infections with ozone therapy.

The patient is connected to an infusion arrangement and blood flows into the bag. This blood is subjected to carefully calibrated concentration of ozone which is rich in oxygen. When the blood is exposed to ozone it becomes saturated with oxygen. The blood is infused back into the patient's circulation.

The procedure can be repeated several times in a single therapy session. It is claimed that as many as ten passes have been successfully carried out safely in a single treatment session.

Dr. Frank Shallenberger's clinic in Reno and Dr. Al Sears in Palm Beach, Florida also offer hyperbaric procedures to increase oxygen in your circulation.

Dr. Shallenberger teaches other health professionals, mostly holistic practitioners, on how to administer intravenous ozone. You can google to find a practitioner in your area.

Getting ozone is equivalent to putting jet fuel in your combustion engine. With proper training, intravenous ozone/hydrogen peroxide can be safely administered.

If you know that you are going to have major surgery, and you have enough time, you might prepare by having pre-conditioning ozone therapy before having the surgery. This reduces incidence of post surgical cardiac and renal ischemic reperfusion injury.

Oxygen medicine is more commonly practiced in Europe. It is freely taught and used in Cuba. The FDA has gotten involved in the USA and it is not commonly practiced here. It is not illegal, but you have to go hunting for its availability. And absorb it's cost from private resources. Health insurance does not cover its cost since it is not approved as part of commonly accepted standard practice.

To recap: the oxygen taken in from your breathing must meet the nutrients at the mitochondria. Then at their ideal pH, the Krebs biochemistry works its magic of making the ATP which sustains life.

ELECTRIC MEDICINE

Living humans need to maintain an electric potential in every part of their body.

Your heart beat is sustained by an electrical voltage. Your brain creates electrical function measured by E.E.G. To perform a test of life is to measure the electrical activity of the brain. A flat line EEG means you can be declared medically and legally dead.

Your heart broadcasts a much stronger electric field than your brain. It is measurable with the right equipment.

We will continue this line of thought in the section on the electric body.

CHOLESTEROL AND FATS

Complications of diabetes if allowed to go unchecked, result in multi system disease. Perhaps you could look at diabetes as a micro vascular abnormality. Blood goes to the furthest reaches of the body through the vascular system. Oxygen and nutrients are transferred across cell cytoplasm and cell walls to the interstitial fluid that fills the spaces around cells. Good healthy cell walls facilitate this exchange.

High circulating glucose levels are toxic to the endothelium of capillary vessels. This is especially disastrous in the eyes. It is the one place in your body where an opthalmologist can look directly at blood vessels in real time. Diabetics need to be examined regularly by an opthalmologist to look for diabetic retinopathy.

Two major complications of diabetes are cataract formation in the lens of the eye and retinal hemorrhages, which if severe enough could lead to blindness. Fortunately opacified cataract lenses can be removed surgically and new artificial lenses are inserted. Some of the lenses have built in diffraction prescription so that you may not need to wear glasses after cataract removal.

Diabetics are especially vulnerable to small vessel disease in the extremities, especially the feet. A significant number of amputations occur in diabetics. They have poor blood supply to the skin and soft tissues. Ulcerations occur, and heal slowly or poorly or not at all. In extreme cases, patients with diabetes need access to hyperbaric oxygen facilities. Intravenous ozone/oxygen is also helpful.

AVAZZIA protocols have been developed to accomplish rapid healing of diabetic ulcers, soft tissue wounds and scar tissue. Micro-electric current is applied.

Oxygen travels down a pressure gradient from lung to mitochondria. Numerous cell walls and membranes must be crossed on that journey.

You need healthy cell walls to facilitate that journey. Cell walls are made up of the lipids and cholesterol so your diet needs to supply good fats. Essential fatty acids and cholesterol are necessary for membrane health.

There is a myth that cholesterol is dangerous to your health and associated with cardiac disease. This has never been proven scientifically and needs to be totally eliminated from the any consideration of heart disease.

In fact the scientist who started the myth of connecting cholesterol to cardiac disease was not even a medical doctor. How that came to pass is a story for another place and time. It involves complicated congressional politics.

You need cholesterol. If you completely avoided eating foods containing cholesterol, your liver would make cholesterol during the night when you're asleep in obedience to circadian rhythms. There is no such thing as good cholesterol and no bad cholesterol. The only dangerous cholesterol is oxidized cholesterol.

Eggs have acquired a false reputation as a source of dangerous cholesterol.

In fact, eggs are a complete protein, and good for you. Especially organic eggs. And especially the yolk.

When cholesterol is fractionated, it is found to exist in different particle sizes and molecular weights. Particles exist as large fluffy low density particles, low density particles (LDL), extra-low density particles, and smaller high density particles.

Low density particles LDL are usually calculated ... not counted, unless you do a NMR particle count.

LDLs are carriers of cholesterol. LDL itself is not a primary abnormality. Your LDL is a carrier molecule that transports cholesterol from the liver where it is produced, to wherever it is needed to be incorporated into cell walls, and brain tissue. LDL is the carrier taxi, and cholesterol is the passenger. If some of the taxis are empty, the LDL count will not reflect the number of cholesterol particles. There will be a numerical mismatch.

The smaller high density particle has a damaging effect on endothelial cells of blood vessel lining. Endothelial damage results in plaque formation which is actually an attempt to heal the endothelial damage. If there is a large number of the small high density particles it is a potential source of vascular disease. HDL (high density lipoprotein) is called good cholesterol but this is not 100% correct. Smaller HDL particles are inflammatory but the larger HDL particles are benign and recirculate cholesterol back to the liver.

If your test for fractionation shows a predominance of the large fluffy, low density particles, you are relatively safe from heart disease regardless of your total cholesterol, if even it is elevated.

A good test for cholesterol investigation is to get a Nuclear Magnetic Resonance particle profile.

Regular lipid tests are not good enough to give you the information you really need. They are cheaper, but fall short in critical information.

Your own health plan may be more interested in keeping costs down, than in obtaining the information you should have for effective care.

A rough check of your susceptibility to cardiac disease is to look at your HDL to triglyceride ratio. If the ratio is less than 3, you have a low risk of heart disease.

There are a few exceptions for some hereditary lipid disorders. Cholesterol is necessary for vitamin B complex formation and cholesterol maintains healthy nerve sheaths. Diabetics may suffer from burning pains and tingling of hands and feet. Vitamin B complex is necessary for healthy nerves. Overall vitamin and mineral nutrition must be maintained.

Statin drugs interfere with the chain of events that would wind up in the manufacture of cholesterol and CoQ10 at two different important steps. One is interruption of CoQ10 formation which is crucial for cardiac energy production. A greater harm is done by taking statins, for a lesser benefit of unnecessarily reducing cholesterol, and placing you at a greater risk of heart failure by interrupting CoQ10 formation.

If you do take a statin, then you must absolutely compensate by consuming CoQ10 supplement which is fat soluble. So take it with some healthy fat. e.g. coconut oil MCT, grass-fed butter, flax oil, ghee, or Panaseeda oil.

Amazingly, in this day and age of freely available scientific information, you still see recommendations advising you to take statins.

These recommendations come from government approved bodies. And prominent doctors whose personal reputation is used to justify continued use of statins. This is an attempt to make it conform to good medical practice guidelines that all doctors follow.

Even if your doctor believes whatever new information you give him, he/she is unlikely to use it to provide care for you as an individual. Your doctors could be sued for malpractice if they deviate from "good practice community standard" as listed by licensing authorities. If your doctor follows community standards he/she is held harmless (not guilty) if accused of malpractice.

The latest stab in the dark about statin use, is that it MIGHT have a beneficial effect in Alzheimer's disease.

A report from Cleveland Clinic in July 2015 claims that men on statins have a 46% increased chance of developing diabetes.

Just because a doctor is a recognized authority in one medical specialty, is no reason for you to transfer his/her expertise proclaiming the benefits of statins.

Big Pharma is not giving up easily to keep the statin cash-cow alive and well.

There is an observation that states:

> "Newer concepts in medicine will not be put into practice, till the present generation of doctors all die out. The present generation is stuck with 'standard of care'. A new generation of doctors who have had modern advances taught to them in medical school will result in better care." Max Planck is reported to have said: "Science advances one funeral at a time."

Current news is beginning to advocate statins as a preventive measure. If even you don't already have any signs or symptoms, it is recommended that you should take statins to prevent new plaque formation.

To follow this advice, everybody will be on cholesterol watch. Just think of the financial bonanza for Big Pharma.

How government became involved in the cholesterol recommendations is a story for another time and place. If you follow the latest recommendations, the whole world will soon be taking statins.

Consumer beware!!

What form of fatty acids do you need to take? Some of them can be manufactured by the body. Others cannot. You must add the essential fatty acids which you need in the form of supplements.

Fats exist as long chain fatty acids, medium chain fatty acids and short chain fatty acids. Humans thrive best on medium chain (MCT) and short chain fatty acids. They occur naturally in human breast milk. These shorter chain fatty acids bypass the triglyceride metabolic pathway and go directly to the liver where they are burned for energy. They do not contribute to increasing body fat.

You need Omega 3 fatty acids and Omega 6 fatty acids with a proper balance of 3 : 6. Ideally there should be 2 or 3 of sixes to each Omega 3. Best of all would be a 1 : 1 ratio which is extremely difficult to obtain. Flax oil and macadamia nut oil are excellent sources of Omega 3 fats.

If you supply essential fatty acids, your body will take the raw material and incorporate them into healthy cell membranes that permit the easy transfer of oxygen and nutrients on their way to the mitochondria.

To repeat:

You need omega 3 fatty acids, omega 6 fatty acids and a smaller amount of omega 9 fatty acids. The best ratio of omega 3 to omega 6 is 1 : 1 or 1 : 2

An overabundance of Omega 6 has crept into modern diets. Our modern dietary intake upsets this ratio by as much as 20 times Omega 6, to 1 of omega 3.

You need to monitor your fat intake carefully.

Why?

Because the wrong excess results in inflammation. Chronic inflammation is a basic cause of disease in the body. If you could eliminate chronic inflammation you could eliminate many or all disease. CRP test (C-reactive protein) is a marker for inflammation. Homocysteine is another marker for inflammation. You need the sensitive-CRP test. Not the regular routine CRP test.

So your fat intake is crucial. Be specially attentive to the quality of fat that you consume.

Where can you find Omega 3 essential fatty acids?

The very lowest species of unicellular phytoplankton in the ocean produces Omega 3. Plankton is consumed by krill. Krill is consumed by smaller fish. Smaller fish are consumed by larger fish. Eventually whales consume sea life by the tons. As the fish size increases, the probability of contamination with toxic chemicals increases. So large fish as a source of Omega 3 is less desirable. Solution is to extract fish oil from deep ocean fish. An exception might be cod liver oil from deep ocean fish in clean waters. Krill oil and calamari oil are safe.

Omega 3 comes as:

> EPA (eicosapentaenoic acid)
>
> DHA (docosahexaenoic acid) and
>
> ALA (alphalinolenoic acid).
>
> DHA is the main structural component of your brain.
>
> EPA is considered to be inflammatory.
>
> ALA comes mainly from plant sources and is not easily usable by humans.

DHA can actually react with photons from sunlight and create direct electrical current. You momentarily become a solar cell. Plus you create Vitamin D. No wonder being in the warmth of the sun feels so good.

Fish oil ratio of EPA to DHA is suboptimal. Omega 3 from algae is best.

The best situation is to provide the body a supply of essential fatty acids and let your body assemble the lipids it needs. Like providing a construction worker with enough construction materials and letting him use whatever is needed to erect a building (your body).

There is actually a product called OCEANS ALIVE which is grown from two specially selected species of phytoplankton in huge vats. This is as low as you can start in the food chain to get your essential fatty acids.

Source of Oceans Alive is: Activation Products of Canada. CEO is Ian Clark.

Marine based omega 3 is preferable to plant based omega if you can get it.

Oceans Alive is a green superfood. It is a two-strain algae complex. It has the highest Superoxide

Dismutase of any organism on earth. It has X3200 the antioxidant power as Vitamin C.

Chlorella and spirulina are recommended because of their high nucleic acid content. Fermented chlorella is now available. This is true, but neither chlorella nor spirulina is part of a natural food chain.

To repeat: chlorella and spirulina are not part of a natural food chain. They are cultivated in large lakes.

LIVER

You'll need a healthy functioning liver to be in good health. There are multiple metabolic functions performed by the liver. It is intimately involved in handling insulin, glucose, fats, cholesterol and glycogen. It produces bile which is stored in the gallbladder.

When the body's circulating triglyceride level is increased, the liver can be used as a fat storage depot. Fatty liver infiltration results in a poorly functioning liver. It is necessary to our detoxify the liver in order to return it to good health.

Silymarin (milk thistle) and Bergamot citrus extract are good detoxification agents to cleanse the liver. Bergamot extract reverses non-alcoholic fatty liver disease. NAFLD. Fasting clears the liver and pancreas of fatty infiltrates to restore insulin sensitivity.

Accumulation of fat in the liver and pancreas contribute to the development of insulin resistance. The liver is the single organ that performs more necessary jobs than any other organ in the body. It is also the only organ that regenerates itself. If you remove a big piece of liver to donate for a transplant, it will grow back to its original size. It is currently the only organ which has the capacity to regrow a significant volume of tissue.

NUTRITION, EXERCISE AND SLEEP

A healthy body needs fats, carbohydrates, proteins, vitamins, minerals, clean water, a supply of oxygen, and enzymes that are working at a pH of 7.2 or slightly higher. Total metabolic function results in a production of energy and warmth.

Warmth is a reflection of good thyroid metabolism. If you have low thyroid function you are likely to feel cold all the time. The best form of thyroid supplementation is nascent iodine which is elemental iodine. The biological production of ATP is not 100% efficient. What is lost generates heat, and hence body warmth. The body also needs to be in electrical balance. That is why doctors order metabolic electrolyte test panels. To check your electrical status.

Exercise increases vascular endothelial cells functionality of producing nitric oxide. This relaxes blood vessels and lowers blood pressure.

Nitric oxide is the basis of how Viagra works (see unrelated diversion).

The best form of exercise is High Intensity Training. Short periods of intense exercise, followed by longer periods of rest give the best performance benefits. During exercise, the endothelial cells of blood vessels make and release nitric oxide. This increases delivery of oxygen to tissues.

Long hours of gym exercise is less useful than short bursts of high intensity exercise.

Dr. Al Sears offers his PACE PROGRAM that outlines how to do high intensity training. Dr. Sears owns and operates the Sears Institute of Antiaging Medicine in Florida.

His Progressive Accelerating Cardiovascular Exertion program P.A.C.E. takes 12 minutes to do a complete cycle of high intensity training. It emphasizes improvement of lung capacity and cardiac endurance.

Another form of exercise is VARIABLE INTENSITY INTERVAL EXERCISE. It consists of a mixture of low intensity, medium intensity and high intensity segments. There is a combination of mind-body exercise, strength and agility exercise and high intensity exercise.

If you are physically unable to exercise, you might try vibration plates. These provide the same benefits of regular gym exercise without the strenuous physical exertion. These machines provide vertical and horizontal vibrations, or combination of movements. You stand on a platform, set your program and timer, and away you go.

Even wheelchair bound people can use vibration plates. Vibration plate exercise is very good at stimulating the flow of lymphatic fluid.

One good choice of vibration platform is HYPERVIBE 17 but you only have to do a computer search to find many others. Pick your price. Pick a vibration plate.

Dr. Yoshiaki Sato of Japan has devised an exercise system that gives similar benefits as high intensity training without the strenuous exertion. His research started in 1966. His system is called KAATSU TRAINING. It is used successfully in professional sports. Professional football teams, Olympic athletes and body builders have been applying this training.

The basics of the system depends on restriction of venous blood flow back to the heart. Compression bands are wrapped around the proximal arms and legs. Arterial blood flows through but surface venous flow is interrupted. At the same time as the venous return is delayed, while exercising, smaller weights are used compared to regular weight training, and the number of repititions are increased. The combination is less stressful physically than HIT.

Because venous blood remains longer in the muscles, lactic acid is increased. This fools the brain into thinking that intense workout is in process. It triggers increased mTOR signals and down-regulates myostatin gene expression. Myostatin suppresses muscle growth. Down-regulation promotes muscle growth.

KAATSU stimulates muscle growth and strength with lower physical exertion. There is also less liablity to injury. In effect, you get the same rewards as for high intensity exercise.

UNRELATED DIVERSION

Just as nitric oxide produces vasodilation, nitroglycerine produces vasodilation. So too does cayenne extract. You should keep some cayenne in your emergency kit. It has a long half- life before losing potency. If someone needs nitroglycerine at short notice, and none is available, try using cayenne extract till you can get to an emergency room. It should produce vascular dilatation till effective medical help is available.

INFLAMMATION

Inflammation is ever present in the background, keeping a constant vigil over our well-being. When our ancestors moved from the trees to existence on the ground, they became exposed to injuries, cuts, fractures, pierced skin and infections etc. It became an evolutionary necessity that we develop the process of inflammation. We experience redness, heat, swelling, pain and loss of function. Acute inflammation is necessary to cure short term illnesses. And then turn itself off. If it continues beyond that point, it becomes chronic inflammation. Acute inflammation is good and desirable. Chronic inflammation is bad and undesirable.

Chronic inflammation has been blamed for being the cause of all curable diseases.

PROTEINS

Proteins are necessary to build new tissue in every organ system. Replacement of worn out tissue must occur. It is estimated your entire body structure is replaced on an average of every six to twelve months.

Every cell in your body has been replaced in the last year or so. Various time intervals appear in the medical literature, but one year is a good broad range.

Metabolically, you are no more than a year old.

Some cells are replaced in days or weeks. These rapidly replaced ones are the ones affected most quickly by chemotherapy in cancer patients. Others get replaced more slowly. Examples are bones and enamel of your teeth. Your entire skeleton and teeth may take as long as five to seven years to be replaced. One thing is certain. The human body is constantly being regenerated.

What is currently under investigation is whether the new cell population is a copy of a previously existing old cell or a brand new one generated by new stem cells.

There has been a recent rash of claims that you can take a magic pill, and regenerate your entire body with new, young cells derived from stem cells that already exist in a dormant state in the body.

Unfortunately, these rosy claims are short on details but encourage you to buy immediately. You have to buy larger amounts to get the best price. Most of them are about the same price, so there must be some form of collusion and price fixing.

Current investigation explores the significance of telomeres and stem cells.

The philosophical hunt for longevity asks the question of why we grow old. Why do we get diseased? Can we have a longer and healthier life? Hayflick Limit says that there is a finite number of cell divisions and basically determines how long we can live. Is there a limit to the number of replications? Can these be reversed? Whenever cells divide, the telomeres at the end of chromosomes become shorter.

Eventually telomeres become progressively shorter till the Hayflick limit is reached and tissues progress to death.

Fortunately, there is an enzyme called telomerase which lengthens telomeres.

If longer telomeres extend the life of cells we might get immortal cells, which is what cancer cells are. They have unlimited and unregulated growth. So we need a balance between too much and too little mTOR activity.

The use of telomerase supplements is still under investigation.

How much protein do you need daily? Can you supply pre-digested amino acids and let the body assemble what it needs? Can you get the necessary amino acids as supplements or do you need to eat real food. Your body matrix is held together with collagen and vitamin C which is essential for adhesiveness of tissue. Remember scurvy?

Parent essential fatty acids include Omega 6 and Omega 3 essential fatty acids.

Fats provide energy. Fats release 9 calories of energy for each gram consumed as compared to 4 calories per gram of carbohydrates or proteins. Fat is more energy efficient.

You can consume less fats to get more calories. You can therefore eat less to produce the same amount of energy.

Fats satisfy your hunger more quickly than carbohydrates and for a longer period of time.

There is a constant conversation going on between your brain and your stomach. Hormones such as ghrelin and leptin are the mediators.

A DEEPER LOOK AT PROTEIN METABOLISM

mTOR is an ancient signalling pathway found in virtually all organisms including bacteria.

mTOR gene is located on chromosome 1.

mTOR stands for measured target of rapamycin. Formerly called mammalian target of rapamycin. That is why it was originally called mTOR. It is now known to apply to all living things, not only to animals.

mTOR is regulated by protein intake. More protein intake increases the amount of mTOR. mTor regulates the activity of insulin, leptin, and growth factor (IGF). It governs metabolism, growth, cell differentiation and cell survival. It governs removal of cell detritus from senescent cells.

mTOR decides if cells should replicate now, or stay alive to replicate later. It regulates autophagy. Damaged mitochondria are removed along with cell debris.

As mTOR increases, autophagy decreases. Intermittent fasting turns off the mTOR gene. When it is overactive it is associated with early mortality, cancer and Alzheimer's disease. At any one time, there is competition between regeneration of tissue and breakdown of tissue. If we could repair damage as fast as it happens, perhaps we could live forever, or at least a very much longer time than the proverbial three score and ten.

Constant mTOR activation should be avoided. It works best if you alternate between mTOR stimulation and and intermittent fasting which down-regulates mTOR activity. This way, you alternate protein build up, and removal of dead or dying cell debris.

To do this, reduce unlimited protein intake. Estimate half a gram of good quality protein for each pound of lean body mass. Maximize at 40 - 70 grams daily.

No more than 25 grams of protein in your largest meal. It is well known that calorie restriction will extend your lifespan. Pig out now and die sooner or restrict calorie intake and live longer. Take your pick.

Is there an easier way out? Look at supplements that mimic low mTOR activity. Two examples are TELO-SC from Maxlife and oxaloacetate. TELO-SC is an mTOR inhibitor.

Oxaloacetate works in the background. Take the supplement and leave your lifestyle undisturbed. Your normal cells produce oxaloacetate in the Krebs cycle of ATP generation. Supplements can accelerate this function. Among other things, oxaloacetate suppresses mTOR. This increases autophagy. It has the same effect as caloric restriction, hence it increases longevity.

Since oxaloacetate functions the same as calorie restriction, a bonus is that weight loss occurs gradually when you take the daily supplement. No dieting necessary.

Which circles back to an environment that is hostile to the development of cancer.

There is progressive accumulation of evidence that cancer is primarily a mitochondrial disease. One book is included in the short reading list: TRIPPING OVER THE TRUTH. It expands on the concept of cancer as a mitochondrial disease.

Another useful supplement is niacinamide riboside, a Vitamin B3. It functions as a niacin, without the hot flush that accompanies niacin intake. Niacin flush is an undesirable side-effect. It can be avoided by taking nicotinamide-riboside instead of plain niacin.

Niacinamide is readily converted to bioactive NAD+ (nicotinamide adenine dinucleotide) which is involved in the Krebs cycle and helps to regenerate ATP.

Hormone messages between the brain and the stomach govern the feeling of hunger. Therefore you need to eat fats to get a feeling of fullness for a longer period of time. Carbohydrates do not provide this benefit.

The double membranes that make up the walls of your individual cells are dependent on a good supply of essential fatty acids and cholesterol. You need to be careful about the quality of food that you eat. Dietary intake of fats include molecules comprised of short chain fats, moderate length chain fats and long chain fats. The basic structure of a fat is a central unit, to which side chains of various elements are bonded. These bonds may be unsaturated and will have room for more chains. Saturated, polyunsaturated, and saturated fats are just examples of fats. Some exist as solid. Others are semisolid at room temperature and others are liquid.

A great deal of information is floating in the medical literature about healthy fats. Suffice it to say that some are better for you to consume and others are detrimental to your health. You need to avoid transfats altogether. Despite the enormous commercial hype and totally misleading information that pervades the commercial world you need to understand what kind of fats to consume. Reliable data must be carefully screened.

As a diabetic you need to consume the best fats you can get.

Your body chemistry has an enzyme switch (AMPK enzyme pathway). Adenosine Activated Protein Kinase. It governs whether you are a fat- burner or a fat storer. A sugar- burner or a fat-storer.

Unused sugar is converted to fat for storage.

AMPK flips the switch between AMPD (deaminase) and AMPK (kinase).

If the switch flips in the direction of AMPD, fat synthesis is increased and insulin resistance is increased.

If the switch flips in the direction of AMPK, fat burning is increased, and you become more sensitive to insulin.

There is recent evidence that metformin taken by diabetics may boost the action of AMPK. The

FDA has approved a study to investigate the use of Meformin as an anti-aging drug.

There are other benefits of metformin. AMPK facilitates DNA repair. It reduces the incidence of cancer. Metformin has been in use for a long time and is a relatively safe drug for widespread use.

Research at Auburn University revealed that circumin in turmeric is 400X more potent than metformin in activating AMPK, an enzyme that plays an important role in glucose transport. Circumin increases insulin sensitivity which can help reverse type 2 diabetes.

Circumin reduces inflammation. It protects against diabetic neuropathy and retinopathy. It reverses insulin resistance and lowers blood sugar. Turmeric has become a natural treatment of choice.

Circumin is fat-soluble and absorption is increased with the addition of bioperine from pulverized black-pepper. Optimally you need both some fat and some bioperine.

The benefits of circumin in turmeric was recognized by the University of California which reportedly tried to file a patent application with the U.S. Patent Office. The government of India dissuaded them from granting a patent because turmeric has been used as a folk remedy in India for thousands of years.

Circumin kills cancer stem cells. These are the ones which are responsible for the recurrence of cancer.

Primary chemotherapy kills current cancer cells but leave the stem cells behind. Circumin kills the surviving stem cells.

Insulin is a fat storage hormone. If you eat fats and carbohydrates at the same time you confuse your body. What should I do with this supply of carbohydrates, burn it for energy or store it as fat? Carbohydrates and sugar (glucose) can be burned immediately for energy or stored in muscle tissue or stored in the liver as glycogen. Or stored as fat. Any carbohydrate not burned immediately is converted to triglyceride and stored as fat.

You have enough carbohydrate to last a few days if subjected to starvation. Fat storage is enough for you to subsist for a few weeks if subjected to starvation. Witness the appearance of people who survive in concentration camps. When carbohydrates and fats are depleted, proteins begin to be consumed. Cachexia sets in. As a diabetic you need to watch closely everything that you eat.

As a diabetic you need to watch closely everything that you eat. How much you eat. What you eat. When you eat it. And what you eat together in the same meal. Never eat fats and starches at the same time. Eat fruits up to half an hour before significant protein consumption or wait till two hours later.

There are fat diabetics and there are skinny diabetics. Are you fat because you are a diabetic first and then became fat or did you become fat first and that led to your becoming diabetic secondarily?

Round and round it goes. Like which came first, the chicken or the egg.

Carbohydrates get digested to glucose which is a sugar. Insulin facilitates the transfer of glucose from the circulation into tissue cells. This transfer occurs across the cell walls. If this is prevented because of insulin resistance, it means that glucose levels in the plasma increases.

This elevated glucose is toxic to the body and cascades into damage to vessels, organs, eyes, kidneys, heart, gut and nerves.

The brain uses glucose as its primary source of energy but it can also use ketones from fatty acids for energy.

If glucose is unavailable the brain will happily exist on ketones from fat metabolism.

SLEEP

Sleep is a necessity. Humans require sufficient restful sleep for good brain health. You need to sleep in complete darkness if possible. Turn off electric appliances in your bedroom. Electric blankets, alarm clocks, night lights. Anything that glows. If you must have a nightlight, make it one that has amber spectrum, not blue or white. Amber light does not disrupt your sleep cycle if you have to get up for a bathroom visit.

The brain goes into anabolic state during sleep. It restores the immune system, nervous system and muscular systems. During sleep there is glympathic clearance of interstitial metabolic waste in the brain. The space between your brain cells increases in size, allowing the interstitial spinal fluids to move more freely, and washing out metabolic waste.

The glymphatic system is most efficient when you are sleeping on your side. Not when you are sleeping on your back or on your tummy.

You should try and sleep on your right side if possible. The glymphatic clearing of intracerebral waste is enhanced.

In addition, when you lie on your right side, the heart is on your upper left half. It is easier for your heart to pump blood "downstream" to the lower right side. If you were lying on your left side, the heart would work harder to perfuse your upper right side.

Be kind to your heart.

In addition, the pyloric outlet of your stomach faces the right side of your body (unless you have situs inversus). It means that gastric secretions do not collect in your stomach while you are asleep. It greatly reduces the chances of your having gastric reflux if you do have a hiatus hernia.

The 2017 Nobel prize in Medicine was just awarded to the researchers who discovered the molecular mechanism that govern circadian rhythms.

Sleep is governed by circadian rhythms. There are two major drivers of the urge to sleep. One is the circadian rhythm that lasts roughly for one whole day. This was established by Nathaniel Kleitman and Bruce Richardson (U. of Chicago) The cycle is split into roughly 15 hours of waking and 9 hours of sleep. Start of waking cycle is triggered by sunrise which shuts off the production of melatonin. Any bright light will accomplish the same thing. E.g. bathroom light.

Darkness signals the start of the sleep cycle. First thing that occurs is the lowering of your body core-temperature by about 1 degree Celsius. Next the pineal gland starts to secrete melatonin for a few hours and this secretion is terminated by light of any intensity. Hence the need to sleep in complete darkness. Use a sleep mask if necessary.

The second driver of the urge to sleep is accumulation of adenosine. The body has a supply of adenosine triphosphate, adenosine diphosphate and adenosine monophosphate to supply adenosine for the sleep cycle. There is continuous accumulation of adenosine as the day progresses, and peaks by sunset.

Circadian rhythm and adenosine concentration work in tandem but are independent of each other.

Adenosine is used up during the night and declines steadily. Glymphatic clearance washes it out of the brain at night. The cycle starts out again the next morning.

Adenosine sleepiness can be blocked by caffeine which competes with it for receptor sites. The half

-life of caffeine is about seven hours. It is cleared by the enzyme P450 1A2 in the liver.

nonREM sleep and REM sleep are important for consolidating memory. During early sleep, nonREM predominates and during later sleep, REM dominates.

During REM sleep brain electrical activity is very prominent, but this is accompanied by a concurrent paralysis of voluntary muscles. Memories are transferred from the hippocampus to the prefrontal cortex for permanent storage. Consolidation of permanent memory requires a few days, hence the advice to "sleep on it".

This consolidation of memory is relevant to Alzheimer's Disease which is manifested with loss of memory. Adequate sleep is crucial to getting nonRem and Rem sleep in synchrony to increase your memory bank.

The urge to sleep is intensified by sleep deprivation. Extreme sleep deprivation could result in involuntary episodes of microsleep. You lose concentration. You lose vision. You lose motor control. If you experience an episode of microsleep while driving in heavy traffic, it could be the end of your life.

There are sleep disorders to consider, but they are not included in this book.

The gene for circadian rhythm and sleep timing is located at Chromosome 12. You have 46 pairs of chromosomes. Half of them come from each parent.

The circadian governing center is located at the supra-chiasmatic nucleus of the brain, just above the optic chiasm, where the optic nerves cross on their way from each eye to the opposite cortex of the brain.

Two major kinds of sleep are REM sleep and non-Rem sleep. As one drifts into sleep, the eyes have a tendency to roll around gently. This is Rapid Eye Movement sleep. R.E.M.

Circadian Cycle is the inner timing clock. This clock is based on external light signals.

With the onset of darkness, the brain produces the hormone melatonin which makes you sleepy. Tryptophan is converted to serotonin and this goes on to end up as melatonin.

You sleep in cycles. You don't simply fall asleep and then wake up several hours later when it is time to get out of bed and be ready for a new day.

A complete sleep cycle lasts from 70 to 90 minutes. A whole night is taken up by four to five sleep cycles. Time-wise that is 360 to 450 minutes.

REM cycles repeat approximately 90 minutes apart. Newborns spend about nine hours in REM sleep. Adults are in total REM sleep for much less time. Adults need six to seven hours of sleep. Eight or more hours is associated with increased mortality.

As you drift into sleep the brain's electrical activity goes from beta frequency 20 + Hz, or higher, to alpha frequency 8 - 13 Hz, next to theta frequency 4 - 7 Hz and finally into delta frequency of less than 3.5 Hz. Progressively slower.

As the frequency decreases you go deeper and deeper into sleep. Slow wave sleep is most restful. Delta sleep is most restful of all.

This is when the brain releases neuro-endocrine hormones. You need to sleep long enough to experience an optimal number of sleep cycles. Hence you need to get into bed early enough.

If you have trouble falling asleep, you could listen to delta frequency music for a short period before retiring for the night. Your brain becomes attuned to the lower frequency and enables you to go to sleep faster instead of staying awake for hours.

You experience several sleep cycles and sometimes wake up and go back to sleep. Various states of arousability occur, depending on which frequency of Hz you are in, at any specific time.

You could be "dead to the world" or you could be in a state of light sleep and easily awakened. You feel refreshed if you wake up as you transit to a new cycle. If you are awakened in the middle of a cycle, you feel that something is not right.

If you take naps during the day, you need to keep the nap shorter than a complete cycle. If not, you disturb your regular circadian rhythm.

SLEEP HACKING is not for the faint of heart. It involves the application of trans-cranial electricity to influence the brain so that you could sleep for fewer hours daily (maybe 3 or 4) and get the same restful effect as having a full night's sleep.

WATER

Second to oxygen, water is the most important nutrition that your body needs. You need clean water for good health. You need good hydration with alkaline pH water to support nutrition.

Electrolytes in water solution move freely around your whole body, carrying nutrition in and waste out and equalizing electricity and desirable pH.

GASTRIC ACID

The pH of the stomach is usually around 2, which is acidic. This acidic barrier protects you from swallowing harmful bacteria. Hydrochloric acid is needed and secreted for digestion.

If you become a hospital inpatient, your physician might routinely prescribe proton-pump-inhibitors which suppress your stomach acid. You lose the benefit of stomach acidity to prevent ingestion of harmful bacteria.

You might want to discuss with your doctor, whether you will get protein pump inhibitor (PPI) routinely or not. Suppression of gastric acid is not normal. If PPI removes the protective acid barrier, you could more easily become infected with Clostridium difficile bacterium that is difficult to treat. Would that meet the criteria of a hospital acquired infection? If so, who is responsible?

Generally when you are admitted to hospital, you are required to sign consent forms that it is possible to get a hospital acquired infection, but the hospital is held harmless.

Catch 22. You are prescribed a PPI which removes the barrier to C.diff, but neither the prescribing physician nor the hospital is responsible.

It is a confirmed fact that taking PPI medication removes the acid barrier and makes you open to ingestion of Clostridium difficile if it is present in your hospital environment.

STRIKE ONE

Normal gastric acidity is around 2.0 pH. Drink enough water to overcome acidity in the stomach, and drink enough volume of alkaline water to make ingested water as a net alkaline solution. You want your net body pH to be alkaline while your gastric pH remains acid. After you have ingested enough water to satisfy your thirst, the stomach will replenish it's acidity again. Avoid drinking water with your meals or you wind up diluting the secreted hydrochloric acid and enzymes that are released for digestion.

You can easily buy Prevacid, Prilosec and Nexium over the counter. These are effective protein pump inhibitors. They stop the production of stomach hydrochloric acid and relieve the symptoms of acid reflux.

Do you really want to do this? Do you know the side effects that you are exposing yourself to? In the first place it is a very bad thing to suppress gastric acid. Hydrochloric in the stomach is necessary, normal and healthy.

You want to prevent backflow into the esophagus. GERD. Gastro Esophageal Reflux Disease.

Reflux is a function of the sphincter at the junction of the esophagus and the stomach. If this sphincter is properly functioning, it will prevent reflux. The presence of gastric acid pH is incidental. What matters is function of the sphincter. Tight sphincter... no reflux. Lax sphincter... reflux.

Suppression of gastric acid is also accompanied by suppression of acids in the lysosomes within microglia cells in the brain. These lysosomes in the brain are responsible for cleaning up beta-amyloid proteins in the brain. Accumulation of beta amyloid influences development of Alzheimer's disease.

Would you really rather risk getting Alzheimer's disease and/or dementia in exchange for some gastric relief? Increased dementia has been documented with prolonged use of PPIs. Moreover treatment for reflux esophagitis can be effectively managed using simpler medical measures. A chewable tablet containing magnesium carbonate, calcium carbonate and a special deglycyrrhized extract of liquorice will protect your esophagus while leaving your stomach pH undisturbed.

Equally important is the proven deleterious effect of PPIs on your kidneys. Acute interstitial nephritis and permanent chronic renal disease as well as renal failure could result from prolonged PPI use. A recent John Hopkins University analysis of 10,000 cases over six years concluded that there was a 35% increase in chronic kidney disease for people taking PPIs over the long term.

STRIKE TWO

PPI use results in an inhibited absorption of Vitamin B12.

Homocysteine levels surge. Together with increased CRP levels. Both are markers of inflammation. There is an increased incidence of osteoporosis and increased incidence of bone fractures. There is increased calcium deposition in coronary arteries.

STRIKE THREE.

PPI is:

Bad for your brains.

Bad for your bones.

Bad for your kidneys.

Bad for your heart.

Wrong treatment for GERD.

TALKING ABOUT WATER

Timing is important.

You should drink water that is enriched with electrolytes. If necessary, you might add drops of fulvic acid to your drinking water. Fulvic acid has electrolytes and micro minerals that you need.

OCEANS ALIVE phytoplankton product achieves the same end result.

You need to consider what you can do with water and the quality of the water you drink. Basic function is to provide adequate hydration so that you get enough fluids to facilitate proper kidney function.

How much water do you need to drink? Enough to have clear urine, and a need to empty your bladder every one to two hours. Sometimes when you have a feeling of hunger, your body is really asking for water.

You will see comments about drinking enough ounces based on your weight. A vague explanation of your body being 70% water really begs the question. It is true, but a non-sequitar.

Your body is about 70% water, roughly ten gallons for an average person. Your bones are about 20% water and even fat is about 25% water. If you slavishly follow those body weight calculations, you run the risk of water intoxication.

You can estimate your water composition by using the right scale to weigh yourself. There are scales that pass a weak electric current through your body and then give you an idea of your body composition in terms of weight of bones, muscles, fat and water.

You have kidneys to regulate your water management.

You maintain healthy hydration which is governed by your glomerular filtration function. If you drink more water than your body needs, the extra water is filtered out by the kidneys.

In addition to alkalinity, consider that you could add electrolytes to the water you drink.

Do not drink distilled water. You need to add back electrolytes or some fulvic acid. You might add oxygen to the water by adding food grade 35% hydrogen peroxide to a dilution that is acceptable to your tastebuds.

Don't forget that you might magnetize the water you drink. Regular tap water, distilled water and bottled water are called "dead water" from a metabolic standpoint. "Living water" comes from a flowing source such as springs and clean running water in streaming rivers.

This water is exposed to spinning vortices that impart "spin" to the water molecules. In nature, there is right spin (dextro rotation) and left spin (levo rotation).

Crystals diffract light in d- and l- directions as you might remember from Chemistry 101.

The DNA water of healthy cells spins to the left. Cancer cell water spins to the right.

Exposing water to scalar energy in a magnetic field produces "living water".

The structure of living water has molecular angle of 109.5 degrees and a closed hexagonal formation. These hexagonal water molecules are smaller and wetter than "dead water", and therefore enter and leave cells more rapidly. This speeds up nutrition and clearance of waste. Also increases oxygenation. "Live water" creates more hydroxyl atoms and tends toward alkalinity. They attract and absorb toxins and flush out the toxins.

Regular non-magnetized water molecules have a 104.5 degree formulation and are mostly pentagonal in composition. The molecules are bigger and a mixture of sizes. They do not flow into and out of cells as readily as smaller hexagonal water molecules. Regular water does not remove toxins which can therefore accumulate inside the cell. The toxins can be absorbed into the water molecule, but becomes trapped inside, and therefore accumulate inside. And maintain your toxic load.

You can add antioxidant molecular hydrogen H2 to your water.

PURATIVE sells Active H2 tablets and Patrick Flanigan sells Megahydrate capsules.

Consider magnetizing the water that you drink.

QuWave sells scalar magnets that magnetize water and produce "live water". Consider oxygenating the water you drink. Consider alkalinizing the water you drink. A pinch of bicarbonate of soda goes a long way.

Dr. Gerald Pollack of University of Washington has discovered that water inside of cells exist in a fourth phase which he calls Exclusion Zone water. It is neither a solid, liquid nor gas phase.

Exclusion Zone is the fourth phase and carries a negative charge. It is critical to the normal functioning of mitochondria inside of cells. If there is not enough fourth- phase water, the cell becomes dehydrated and mitochondria become dysfunctional.

New EZ water is formed spontaneously by exposure to vibration, shaking, exercise, infrared light, and sunlight. Light entering the eyes results in the formation of EZ water.

The use of vibration plates for exercise also benefits you by supplying vibration to create EZ water.

Trampolines also provide vibration to create EZ water and enhance the flow of lymphatic fluid.

The negative charge of EZ is cancelled out by free radicals. Antioxidants reverse this process. The negative charge of EZ water is necessary for the electrical message that cells need to communicate with one another.

COFFEE

A word about coffee since many people make it a prominent part of their ingested liquids. For some people it is their largest intake of daily liquids. It is the most important source of polyphenols in the diet of a vast majority of people.

Green coffee beans are rich in chlorogenic acid. Add one capsule of pure green coffee bean extract to your diet, or whenever you drink a cup of coffee.

Chlorogenic acid helps to prevent glucose spikes in diabetics. It speeds up your metabolism. It suppresses your appetite. It reduces hunger.

Coffee is a stimulant and boosts memory. It is beneficial in modifying neuro-degenerative disease such as Parkinson's and reducing beta-amyloid in Alzheimer's disease.

Caffeine acts as an adaptogen. It increases BDNF. Brain Derived Neurotrophic Factor.

A recent Cardiology meeting in Barcelona shows that coffee drinkers have a 64% decreased risk of dying from any cause, especially over 45 year age group.

Caffeine is an activator of the p3 gene. This facilitates cell apoptosis (scavenging function for removal of dead and/or dying cells). Chronic calorie restriction does the same job, and extends longevity.

Some people do not tolerate caffeine very well. They have genetic variations that cause this intolerance. If you tolerate caffeine well, then you can reap the benefits of drinking coffee. If not, too bad.

There seems to be a constant stream of conflicting reports about coffee. Now it's good for you. Then it's bad for you. Don't believe everything you hear about coffee in the news media.

Sleep might be disturbed by coffee drinking, so you need to balance timing of coffee ingestion. Caffeine stimulates fibrous connective tissues in female breasts, so a mammogram study must be preceded by avoiding coffee for a few weeks before scheduling the mammogram.

Bottom line: There are many benefits for coffee consumption if you tolerate caffeine. Coffee is rich in polyphenols but you must avoid coffee that is contaminated with molds. Remember that if you put milk in your coffee, it binds to the polyphenols and you lose the benefits of the polyphenols.

Lesson: drink "black" coffee. No milk or cream.

Same lesson for tea.

The polyphenols in all tea are called catechins. There are several catechins. The most important one is EGCG. Dairy products bind to the catechins and you lose their benefits. Drink tea without adding milk.

BULLETPROOF COFFEE

Have you ever heard of bulletproof coffee?

How is it different and what can it do for you?

Specific instructions on how to make it can be googled. The guru of bulletproof coffee is Dave Asprey who has written a couple of books on coffee and diets.

Basically you brew coffee or decaffeinated coffee. Add medium chain fatty acids derived from virgin coconut oil. Add small amounts of MCT coconut oil and increase the amount to tolerance level as your gut becomes accustomed to it. If you get ahead of yourself, be prepared to remain close to bathroom facilities in case you have to go in a hurry.

You can avoid this problem if you use ghee (clarified butter) made from the milk of grass fed cows, instead of coconut oil MCT.

You can further improve the nutritional value of bulletproof coffee by adding collagen protein.

Sweeten with ribose or stevia. Ribose is a necessary sugar for ATP production. Ribose is also good for your heart. Turmeric coffee creamer can be found to make your coffee better. LAIRD SUPERFOOD sells several excellent flavored coffee creamers.

You get chlorogenic acid from the coffee, good fats from grass-fed ghee, and amino acids from the collagen.

Bulletproof coffee suppresses your appetite, and you get to stretch out the number of hours that you tolerate hunger before needing to eat. In effect you are getting the benefit of calorie restriction. You are shortening the period allotted for eating, consuming fewer calories and probably losing weight.

A win-win situation all around.

FOOD AND DIETING

If you have been diagnosed with diabetes, it is not the end of the world (though it might feel like it). Eternal vigilance becomes the watchword for the rest of your life. Every morsel of food or liquid that you ingest must be monitored closely and constantly. There is no reward for past good behavior. Only what you do in the present will count in your favor.

Since diabetes is a carbohydrate disorder you know with certainty what you must do.

You must eliminate the vast majority of your carbohydrates. Grains must be eliminated from your diet. Especially wheat. No wheat bread is allowed. Neither whole-wheat bread nor white bread. Other grains are also off-limit.

An exception is sprouted grain bread because sprouted grains are digested as vegetables, not as grains. You could bake your own healthy bread, and control what goes in it. Flour from organic sprouted grain grown hydroponically is available to make your own healthy bread. Avoid wheat and grains of any kind. Sprouted is acceptable substitute.

Get your carbohydrate from fruits and vegetables and nuts. Beans are acceptable. They are rich in fiber and supply vegetable proteins. The quality of protein is not as good as meat proteins.

Avoid all starchy foods. If it is white, don't bite. White cauliflower is an exception, but a variety of "designer organic cauliflowers" is available in several colors.

These will supply glucose when digested. If there is a need for more glucose, the body can generate what you need by a process called gluconeogenesis.

Gluconeogenesis consumes proteins.

This gluconeogenesis is the source of increased fasting glucose as circadian rhythm shifts from sleep mode into awake mode. New glucose is released as the body comes out of sleep and gets ready for a new day. You could possibly wake up with a higher blood glucose level than when you went to bed... all without having had anything to eat.

You will, as a diabetic be able to supply your energy needs by increasing your intake of fats. Good fats include grass-fed butter and ghee, virgin coconut oil, macadamia nut oil, avocado oil, and red-palm oil. They can be used for cooking since they have a high heat smoke point. Virgin olive oil cannot withstand high heat but can be sprinkled on salads. Monounsaturated oils have several unoccupied attachment sites which expose them to oxidation.

You can allot about 40% of your dietary intake to healthy fats without jeopardizing your cholesterol levels and lipid status.

More fat if you follow recommendations by Dr. Mercola. Up to 80 % fat.

Fats make you feel full and supply more energy per unit than carbohydrates. "Butter is better". Try grassfed.

Avoid trans-fats and margarine. Avoid oils made from the seeds of plants. Avoid canola oil. There is no such thing as a canola plant. This oil comes from rapeseed which must be highly processed before being sold as food grade.

Most rape seed has been genetically modified. Numerous studies link canola oil with heart disease, kidney disease and liver disease. Intense marketing has been funded by Canada to make it a popular choice. There is a wide selection of non-controversial products so you can easily avoid consuming canola oil. CANada gave it's name to CANola oil.

Some oil blends are marketed under a disguised false label. Read the labels and you will see as much as 80% of a blend could be canola oil but only 20% of the other oil e.g. grapeseed. You are really buying canola oil under a fake name!!!

Avocados and nuts provide healthy fats.

Macadamia nuts and pine seeds are high in healthy fats.

PROTEINS AND SWEETENERS

Grass-fed meats and organic eggs are good protein choices. Fruits can be incorporated into healthy protein smoothies. Whey concentrates and sprouted grain plant proteins are good choices too. Avoid protein isolates. Use whey concentrates.

Proteolytic enzymes digest extra fibrin in circulation. They clean up metabolic debris.

Proteolytic enzymes decrease blood flow resistance but also lengthens clotting time. Be extra careful if you are on prescription anti-coagulants.

Digestive enzymes act to digest the food we eat as opposed to cleansing functions of those left-over proteolytic enzymes which act to remove extra fibrin floating around in circulation.

You have to drastically reduce adding sugar and sweets to your food.

You have to eliminate soft drinks laced with fructose corn-syrup.

You have to totally eliminate corn syrup and its fructose derivatives.

Stevia is an acceptable sweetener. Honey is OK. Processed agave is bad because of refining procedures. Unrefined agave is probably OK.

Avoid all commercial powdered sweeteners. Some of them are based on rat poison.

WATER AND MINERALS have been covered.

Do not forget to keep an eye on your salt intake as part of your minerals. You need sodium and it usually is taken in as salt. Sea salt and table salt have sodium and chloride as a single molecule. NaCl. Sodium is associated with hypertension. Not everyone is sensitive to sodium, but shotgun medical advice is usually to prescribe for everyone to go on a low salt diet or a salt free diet. Whether you are sodium - sensitive or not.

Nobody ever checks to see if you as an individual actually need to avoid sodium. You really need to have your medical management individualized to you as a separate patient.

Salt restriction could be bad advice because everybody, without exception, needs to have the chloride to make gastric hydrochloric acid for digestion. You may need to take a HCl supplement if necessary.

With increasing age, the stomach becomes less efficient at making HCl. Some people stop making any HCl altogether (achlorhydria) and need to take replacement HCl with their meals on a regular basis.

Wild animals go a long way to find salt-licks to replenish their salt intake.

Remember the PPI problem that suppresses gastric acidity. It is unnatural to be missing HCl in the stomach. You need that acid barrier to prevent yourself from swallowing potentially harmful bacteria.

Unfortunately store bought packaged food is loaded with salt.

Far in excess of what you should be eating. Learn to read labels on prepared packaged food. It totally negates advice to go on a low salt diet if you are consuming store bought processed meals. Best of all is home cooked meals where you can control how much salt is added, and the quality of salt used.

MICROELECTRONICS AND FUTURE MEDICINE

Just ask Nicholai Tesla and Albert Einstein.

TESLA: If you want to find the secret of the universe, think in terms of energy, frequency and vibration.

Everything has electrical frequency or vibrational energy.

EINSTEIN: Everything in life is vibration.

The whole world is one gigantic electrical unit. You are yourself an electrical appliance plugged into the entire system. Energy sustains everything.

Electricity is a form of energy. Electricity exists as charges.

It exists naturally as positive and negative charges. Polar orientations exist. North and south poles exist.

Electricity and magnetism coexist. They are inseparable.

Think of a battery. It has a positive terminal and a negative terminal and a ground. Everything needs to be grounded to a neutral status. The electrical sockets in your house need to be grounded. Electrical equipment needs to be grounded. Working surfaces need to be grounded. Workers using equipment need to be grounded.

The earth is a massive storage reservoir of negatively charged electricity. The upper atmosphere is the location where positive charges accumulate. When the amount of positive charges become large enough, electrical discharge in the form of lightning happens spontaneously and neutral equilibrium is reestablished.

When you accumulate electric negative charges as an individual and you touch a metal door knob, the same thing happens on a tiny scale. Static electrical discharge takes place and you quickly become neutral once more.

There is a big literature on grounding. Grounding mats can be purchased. You can buy grounding bed sheets to sleep on and equalize build-up of electrical charges while you sleep.

You can mentally teach yourself to ground yourself to the center of the earth. The center of the earth is pictured mentally as a large red area at the center of the globe. No matter where you are in the world, your feet are directed to the center of the earth.

Your first chakra at the base of the sacrum is associated with the color red. You ground your first chakra with the negative region at the center of the earth.

Your body is actually an electrical appliance which maintains a millivoltage potential at all times. The cells of your body have a double walled membrane and the ATP energy you produce, maintains a 70 to 90 millivoltage potential across the gap.

This is different from your overall operating voltage of -20 to -35 of millivolts in good health.

When this trans-membrane gradient is disturbed you move from a state of health to a state of disease.

Humans can generate 10 to 100 millivolt potential. You are actually a millivolt electrical generator.

Healing takes place at -50 millivolts according to Dr. Jerry Tennant. He started out in medicine as an Opthalmologist.

There is a correlation of voltage to pH values. On a pH scale of 1 to 14, pH 1 represents the acid end and 14 represents the alkaline end.

Neutral is 7. Your body chemistry functions best at slightly alkaline range of pH 7.3 to pH 7.5. There are charts which show how pH matches voltage. The following limited table shows how micro-voltage corresponds to pH:

0 v. -10	-15	-20	-25	-35
7.0 pH	7.10	7.26	7.35	7.44

VOLTAGE and matching pH below:

In a healthy cell the inside surface membrane is slightly negative to the exterior surface. There are more negative charges on the inside because of a predominance of negative electrolytes on the inside. This is a function of the sodium pump.

Electrolytes are negatively charged and positively charged particles in aqueous solution. They can carry electrical current in water. Cells regulate the passage of electrolytes across membranes. They transport nutrients and waste material in and out of this area as the water moves in and out of the cell.

The electrolytes inside and outside the cells allow a transmission of nerve impulses, contraction of muscles and hormone transport. The presence of electrolytes determines pH. Extra cellular sodium is associated with more positive charges. Potassium is associated with negative charges. Chloride is associated with negative charges. Calcium facilitates muscle contraction.

You are an electric being. That is why your doctor checks your electrolytes when a chemistry panel is performed.

Many processes in the body, especially in the brain and central nervous system and muscles require electrical signals for communication. Sodium is critical in generation of electrical signals. Your body creates electricity to communicate. Flips between negative and positive charges at membranes are responsible for generating electrical impulses.

The earth carries an enormous reservoir of negative charge. It is always electron rich. It supplies an abundant source of antioxidant electrons and free radical busters.

There is constant flow of electric energy between you and the earth when you are in barefoot contact with the earth. You are grounded. You are in resonance with the same negatively charged electric potential as the earth. The earth's resonance frequency is 7.83 Hz and is called Schumann Resonance.

Contact with earth is also called earthing. It is the same as grounding.

Grounding calms the sympathetic nervous system. Grounding supports heart rate variability. Grounding relieves inflammation which is at the root of all disease.

You ground yourself when you walk barefooted on the beach, walk on sand, walk on grass and get into the ocean. Gardening is such a pleasure because you are constantly being grounded as you handle the soil.

But not if you are wearing gloves.

You may buy grounding mats and plug them into a grounded electrical - plug. Be sure to check that the outlet is grounded with a tester you can buy at any hardware or electrical store.

Putting your bare feet on the grounded mat equals walking barefooted as if you are outdoors. It is possible to buy grounding sheets to put on your bed so that you are grounded while you are asleep.

You can practice breathing to ground yourself to the center of the earth if you believe in chakra energy philosophy. You may breathe in through your crown chakra at the center of the top of your head and collect energy at a location just below the navel. From there, you exhale and project energy to the center of the earth. This is your connection to ground.

Next you breathe in and imagine a stream of energy coming up from the center of the earth, through your feet and entering your body again and settling at the so called Dantian, a couple of inches inferior to the navel.

Use your breath to drive energy from your first chakra to the negative center of the earth. Now pull the energy from the grounded site, up into your body and center it at your Dantian. You have grounded yourself.

Repeat a few times. Breathe in. Collect energy at the Dantian. Exhale and project it to the center of the earth. Once the connection is made, reverse the process. Draw the grounded energy up into your feet and let it go back to the Dantian point. You are done. The entire process could take less than a minute.

It happens at the speed of light. You can now get on with the rest of your day.

SUN SALUTATION is a well known yoga practice.

Greet the sun as it rises. Imagine it, if you cannot see the physical sun e.g. if you live in an apartment complex. Face the direction of the rising sun if you cannot see it physically. Install a big sun picture on the wall.

Let it's rays stream directly to the center of your forehead. Let its light and warmth fill your entire being, from the crown of your head to the soles of your bare feet as they touch the ground. (no shoes or socks).

Look to the sun. Imagine its light streaming through your third eye. Center of your forehead. Fill your entire head and body with this light. Imagine this light expanding all around you. One great big ball of light. With you in the center. You are the energy center of the universe. Now dismiss it, and get on with your day.

Dr.Barry Morguelan is a surgeon at University of California at Los Angeles. He is a grand master of Chinese energy medicine.

He has given a detailed explanation of how to perform a meditation of breathing to establish a connection to ground yourself.

The process is similar to the preceding guidance. You pull energy in from your superior chakra, let it go through your body to the center of the earth, go beyond, exit through the opposite crust of the earth, turn around and pierce back and reenter your body into your legs, through your body, beyond the top of your head and exit into the universe.

ELECTRIC ENERGY MEDICINE

In the last few years, electricity is gaining usage for health practices. Medical devices are taking their place in the medical field. The Russian space age started the ball rolling.

You need to be aware of your voltage and vibration frequency.

You can tell where you are on voltage by comparing with your pH.

A healthy human operates somewhere around a frequency range of 62 Hz to 68 Hz.

Extraordinary people operate at higher frequencies. Aim to drag yourself higher.

Sick cells mutate to cancer below 40 Hz.

The process of death begins around 20 Hz to 25 Hz.

Eating meat has a very low frequency level, often below 10 Hz. After all, it has already been dead for a while.

It pulls your operating frequency down/lower.

This could be a plug for vegetarianism.

You can elevate your present frequency level with your diet.

Green smoothies have a frequency of 70 Hz to 90 Hz, depending on what you put in it.

Essential rose oil has a frequency of 320 Hz. Rub some on the soles of your feet.

MICRO ELECTRIC MEDICINE

The age of electric medicine started with the Russian space agency when the question was asked: What if someone became ill or incapacitated in a space station, How would medical assistance be provided?

IN 1989, the FDA and Tulsa University jointly held a conference on emerging electromagnetic medical technology. NASA installed magnetic generators in space vehicles to maintain bone density in astronauts. The FDA has approved electrical treatment for nonunion of bone fractures.

Various electronic devices were being developed by Russia but with the decline of Russian space dominance, the ball was dropped. Funding dried up and the scientists involved drifted way. They eventually migrated to the west.

SCENAR units were developed. Self Controlled Energy Neuro Adaptive Regulator.

AVAZZIA in Texas got FDA approval of hand-held units for treatment of pain without the use of drugs.

Multiple programs have been devised to use it for other conditions, similar to "off label use of approved drugs".

AVAZZIA organizes hands-on practical training through the Academy of Applied Bioelectrophysiology.

Dr. Jerry Tennant of Florida has a biomodulator system using microelectronics, light therapy, pads and hand-held devices.

AWARE sells colored light therapy equipment.

iMRS has units for sale. Prices go up to $6k or more, so you need deep pockets.

iMORE technology uses heart rate variability.

FLEX PULSE BLANKETS are available.

BIOMAT FIR units utilize far infrared heat.

LLL lasers... Low level light lasers have been developed. Different frequencies and different colors are available. Blue light and ultraviolet light are bactericidal. Nasal cannula units have laser light directed to the blood vessels at the base of the brain. The passing blood is exposed to the laser light for therapy. Blood viscosity is reduced, with resultant lowering of blood pressure. Oxygenation is increased. Immune function is facilitated.

INTRAVASCULAR LASER LIGHT therapy is available.

A small catheter with a low level laser light at its end can be inserted into a blood vessel. As the blood flows by, it is exposed to the laser light and absorbs beneficial properties. Your entire blood volume can be exposed if the time is long enough for the procedure.

Intravascular laser light is "invasive", but intranasal Vie Light is a clip-on, with no invasive component. Intranasal units are also much more affordable than PEMF equipment. (Pulsed Electro Magnet Frequency).

When flowing blood is exposed to low level laser light, the chromophores in mitochondria act as photoreceptors for the light and electrons are bumped to a state of higher energy.

Blood flow is increased and inflammation is decreased. The immune system is stimulated. More white cells become available. Lymphocyte B and T cells are increased. More macrophages become available.

Interferon function goes up. Overall, your immune system is stimulated.

The progression of chronic kidney disease is slowed down. This is important because conventional medicine offers very little help in preserving kidney function.

Different colored lasers could be used to fine-tune therapy.

Bioelectric Medicine uses energy in one form or the other. e.g. microelectric currents, light frequency, colors, vibrations, heat and magnetism.

Every tissue and organ in your body has a resonant frequency associated with it. Every tissue has electrical energy and magnetism.

Magnetism is inseparable from electricity.

That is the basis of radiological MRI imaging. No electricity, no magnetism. No magnetism, no MRI.

MRI is one of the miracles of modern medicine. Think of this implication in medicine. Various imaging protocols have been devised. fMRI makes it possible to image functioning of the brain. This is function. Not just anatomy.

If you input a frequency with an external source and it matches the tissue resonant frequency, healing can take place. There have been treatments for Parkinson's disease by exposing the patient's head in a MRI unit. Some measure of success has been reported.

Your body runs on electricity. Life evolved under the influence of the earth's geo-magnetic field. You are in effect an electrical appliance existing in a world of electric energy.

When you visit your doctor, he/she might order an electrolyte panel. This is nothing more than a measure of electrically charged chemicals circulating in your blood. Sodium, potassium, calcium, magnesium, copper, iron, iodine etc. Magnesium is involved in over 300 enzymes systems in a healthy person and iodine is the active mineral in the thyroid that is the master endocrine organ. Nascent iodine is the most usable form of iodine.

Electrolytes carry net electrical charges. Negative and positive charges. These water soluble chemicals are in constant equilibrium, moving into and out of your tissues.

In order to get into or out of a cell, they must cross the cell membrane. That is why you need the right fatty acids available to make cell membranes that facilitate the free passage of electrolytes in water solution. This is how nutrition and oxygen get into cells and how waste is excreted.

A normal healthy cell has an external positive potential with respect to its inner negative electrical status. There is a 'sodium pump' that pushes sodium across a cell membrane. It maintains a balance of three sodium outside the cell for every two potassium inside.

There are channels in the membrane that open up for transfers of calcium and magnesium under the right electrical conditions.

You might have heard of calcium channel blockers for treating hypertension. Beta blockers are also used also for treating hypertension.

EMF (electromagnet frequencies)

They are part everyday life.

Low level EMF is given off by many sources. Electrical power transformers, cell phone towers, microwave transmitters, microwave ovens, cell phones, smart phones, bluetooth, wi-fi and even smart meters in houses are examples of EMF emitters. We live in an ocean of EMF pollution. The levels are unnoticeable but cumulative. You need to pay attention.

There are standards which limit permissible levels of emission, but those standards are unreliable. The regulators often come from the revolving door in which lobbyists and regulators are interchangeable.

EMF is capable of affecting DNA and disrupting mitochondrial function. This damage is caused by disrupting the voltage gated control channels.

EMF overwhelms calcium channels and allows calcium to flood the inside of cells. Normally calcium is kept at a higher concentration outside the cell (usually 1000 outside to 1 inside) and participates in creation of electrical pulses. Calcium is usually pushed back outside after the desired electrical pulse has been created. The massive influx of calcium displaces magnesium from inside the cell. There is normally a delicate balance between magnesium and calcium. They compete for access to the electrically charged channel. If one mineral overwhelms the other, it upsets normal cell electric metabolism.

Modern day cell phones are a big source of EMF. You need to keep cell phones on airplane mode when you are not actually using them. EMF reduces sperm count and motility. Keep laptop computers on a table instead of on your lap. The pacemaker of your heart is sensitive to EMF. Don't store your cell phone in a breast pocket. Use a wired monitor to survey the safety of your sleeping child.

You can use Qu-wave scalar magnets to cancel the bad effects of EMF. Qu-wave magnets can be purchased in various strengths and configurations.

There are whole house units, personal units and even plug-ins to cancel emission from computers and computer monitors.

Cell membranes have surface docking stations to which external molecules attach, prior to their entry into a cell. This is what viruses do. Proper frequency input can change the configuration of cell membranes.

Free radicals are electrically charged and they have to be neutralized by antioxidants to reduce the damage they do to healthy cells.

Some radicals are signalling agents for normal metabolism so there needs to be a delicate balance of their presence. Too many free radicals is harmful. Too little is undesirable. You should not think of totally neutralizing free radicals.

One choice of an excellent antioxidant is chlorine dioxide. Chlorine dioxide has a net negative charge and an alkaline pH.

When chlorine dioxide is absorbed into circulation it has two oxygens as opposed to water which has one oxygen and two hydrogens. Chlorine dioxide hitches a ride on the red cells. Red cells do not discriminate between the oxygen in water and the double oxygens in chlorine dioxide.

Whenever chlorine dioxide meets a positively charged acidic molecule a neutralization reaction takes place. The chlorine dioxide grabs electrons from the positively charged molecule and both of them are annihilated. Positively charged bacteria and viruses are totally destroyed instantly.

Development of antibiotic resistance becomes impossible. Even MRSA bacteria are eliminated. (Methicillin Resistant Staphyloccus Aureus)

As a bonus, chlorine dioxide is short-lived. After about half an hour it degrades into pure water and some harmless salts. You can resume whatever you normally do in your daily routines.

Dr. Jerry Tennant has worked extensively on electricity and the human body. According to him, humans run on electricity. He has developed tables which show how electrical potentials correlate with cell membranes. Every voltage has a corresponding pH value.

Human cells are programmed to operate best between -20 millivolts and -35 millivolts. This corresponds to pH of 7.35 It is also a measure of acidosis and alkalosis.

When your pH status deviates significantly outside a narrow range you are in a diseased condition. To cure this situation you need to rebalance the voltage.

An input of -50 millivolts is healing in essence. The electrical gradient between the inner membrane and outer membrane (double walled cell membrane) of a healthy cell is -90 millivolts. Therapy is aimed at restoring healthy electric potentials. Chronic disease is characterized by low voltages. Therapy is aimed at restoring these low voltages back to higher operating voltages.

Dr. Tennant sells PEMF devices and gives lectures which can be accessed on the internet. Biological Impedance Analysis (BIA) can tell you what your membrane electrical status is.

You can check your pH status with pH Hydrion paper test strips available from internet sources. Salivary pH is an indirect measure of cell voltage. Your urine pH should be lower than your saliva pH.

Your blood plasma is a liquid electrical connection to everything in you, with it's electrically charged chemicals. To be in good health, you need proper nutrition, fiber, proteins, fats, carbohydrates, vitamins, minerals, enzymes, clean water, a generous supply of oxygen, energy, and warmth... all working in a slightly alkaline environment and everything in electrical balance.

You not only have a liquid electrolyte conducting network, you also have a nervous system. Nerves transmit signals by electricity.

There is an additional electrical connection of fascia that is found everywhere in your body. Muscles are wrapped in a thin film of fascia. This fascia conducts electricity. When you have surgery, the incision most likely will disrupt continuity of the fascia. It therefore disrupts conduction of electric signals.

Post- surgical scars develop.

AVAZZIA has protocols for restoring electrical conductivity as well as reducing scars. This might become less of a problem with "keyhole stereotactic surgeries".

AVAZZIA units are frequency generators. Application of inputs is through skin contact using patches, electrodes, and wands. Numerous protocols are available with various frequency settings.

Although AVAZZIA is registered with the FDA for pain management, numerous "off-label" applications exist. Avazzia treatments could help with the opioid epidemic . No drugs used.

Treatments for pain, diabetes, heart disease, renal disease, blood pressure disorders, sciatica, acute trauma, and sports injuries are possible. The entire spectrum of medical conditions is included.

AVAZZIA is nicknamed "doc in a box". You can buy a variety of models, ranging from basic to sophisticated with increasing price quotes. You need deep pockets if you want to go first-class.

Avazzia frequency can be selected to speed up wound healing. Diabetic patients with poor circulation and skin ulcerations that heal poorly, or not at all, can be treated with good success rates. Patients might be able to avoid amputations by having successful treatment with Avazzia units.

Attachments to the frequency generator even avoids direct skin contact when treating skin ulcers and wounds.

Acupuncture meridians are included in possible electro stimulation foci.

The vagus nerve can be stimulated to facilitate parasympathetic activity, thus reducing stress. Since the vagus has branches that spread through the entire body (wandering nerve) it can help to reduce inflammation through the entire body by stimulating one location in the cervical spine region where C 10 exits at the jugular foramen. Bilateral stimulation at the same cervical level is ideal.

A very recent new application of micro-electric medicine relates to cosmetics. Removal of wrinkles takes place by modifying underlying collagen through application of noninvasive electrical current. Basically it is comparable in effect to botox, without needles.

Botox temporarily paralyzes nerves. Microelectronics influences the collagen underlying the wrinkles. Read all about it in CELLULAR MAKEOVER authored by Drs. John & Lorrie Hache.

This applied electricity is of the same order of magnitude as the electrical current generated by the heart.

Hence it's safety.

Solid organs and hollow organs perform electrical functions. Solid organs act as capacitors and hollow organs act as coils in an electric circuit. Solid organs are wired to the back of your body surface, and hollow organs are wired to the front.

The right half of the body is considered to be positively charged. The left side is negatively charged. The anterior half is positive and the posterior half is negative. It is thus possible to assign positivity and negativity to each quadrant.

University of Southern California has received research grants to investigate the application of electricity and magnetism externally and non-invasively to the spinal cord of stroke survivors.

Investigation is aimed at improving the ability of patients to walk. Perhaps they can be returned to mobility. It might even improve incontinence.

The March 2015 issue of Scientific American Magazine front cover is headlined "Electric Cures" with sub heading of: Bioelectronic medicine could create an "off switch" for arthritis, diabetes and even cancer.

The full article is on pages 28 -35 and is written by a neuro-surgeon. (Kevin J. Tracey) It is well worth your reading if you have digital access to archives of Scientific American.

The Wellman Center for Photomedicine at Massachusetts General Hospital is part of the Harvard-MIT Division of Health Sciences and Technology. They are researching the concept of infrared therapy. Photobiomodulation includes lights of all wavelengths.

They start at visible light and extend to near infrared and far infrared spectrum. Near infrared penetrates well into the body. Medically useful therapy requires highly active wavelengths of light that penetrate into deep tissues. You get far infrared energy from infrared heat-lamps and infrared saunas. Higher frequency infrared does not penetrate deeply because it is absorbed by tissue water. Exposure to near-infrared powers the mitochondria to produce additional ATP. Near infra-red light at night produces melatonin and helps you to sleep.

Blue light is particularly good for relieving pain. Red light is good for relieving inflammation.

Kidney failure is basically untreatable medically. Put an array of near-infrared lights where the kidneys are, and it seems to work quite well. Only preliminary work has been done here.

PROBLEM WITH LED LIGHTS

The full story of household lighting remains to be completed.

It is an example of how an advance in LED lighting technology could be having unforeseen complications in health effects.

Sunlight has a spectral range from about 300 nm (nanometers) to 2000 nm and beyond. It includes every conceivable wavelength. Visible light covers from 400 to 780 nm.

LED lights are digital and have discrete spectral peaks. Ordinary white light is continuous, and if split with a prism, you get a rainbow of distribution progressing from red, orange, yellow, green, blue, indigo and violet. ROYGBIV.

LED lights have an excess of blue light but virtually no counterbalancing infrared. LED lights suppress the production of melatonin in the pineal gland and in the retina. It disrupts your sleep. It also down-regulates repair of retinal cells in the eyes. Extended exposure could lead to age related macular degeneration.

LED lights are here to stay. The energy savings are substantial. Soon you will not be able to buy regular bulbs because their manufacture is being phased out.

So what can you do? You can still buy regular incandescent bulbs which are clear and not frosted with white coating. Try to match your bulbs for full spectrum wavelength. After sunset, use blue-blocking glasses to protect your retina.

Dr. Joseph Mercola has published an excellent article on the Health effects of LED lighting in his blog of October 23, 2013.

If you spend a lot of computer screen time, you could do a search for Daniel Georgiev of Bulgaria.

He has written software to manage the radiation that is emitted from computer screens His software is called IRIS. It comes in three versions... basic, mini PRO and PRO.

The basic program is free, and you can invest in miniPro for $5. or PRO for $10. (latest available prices). These are lifetime licenses per computer.

There is valuable information on how you can protect your eyes from the stresses of extended computer use.

Overall, everything is connected to everything else as one big complex electrical network. Your body is that network.

To quote from Current Medicine:

Living Matrix refers to the body as a complete informational system. Containing electrical and electronic components with terms such as conductors, resistors, capacitors and semi-conductors. This Body Electric responds best to electrical and electronic signalling when the right devices are used.

ELECTROPORATION

Have you ever heard of electroporation?

Why might it be of interest to you?

What are plasmids?

If cells are exposed to precisely controlled electricity of known voltage, frequency and intensity, these signals open up temporary nanopores in the bilayered phospholipid walls.

These nanopores fill with water, creating a water-filled hole in a lipid barrier.

Now comes the magic.

A water filled track is created for the passage of plasmids into the cell.

Plasmids are small DNA units in circular formation. Similar to mitochondria. They are little protein factories.

Plasmids can generate proteins, antibodies, hormones, insulin, growth factors, repair or replace genes etc. Replace injectable medications with the help of electroporation. Plasmids can be inserted directly into cells to effect cures.

Electroporation has been used successfully in mice, dogs, pigs, horses and cows.

Can humans be far behind?

You can check WICKIPEDIA for details of what electroporation is, and how it has been applied already in science and medicine.

THE BRAIN

The very essence of you is your brain. It generates electrical signals that can be recorded by an electro-encephalogram. EEG. If you cease to generate EEG signals you are legally dead. Life support can be discontinued. Your main use now is to be an organ donor if you were otherwise healthy.

It is now known that your brain can grow new functional cells under the influence of Brain Derived Neurotropic Factors BDNF. You can develop new functional brain cells with new connections. Most of this growth occurs in the frontal lobe and the temporal lobes. You can grow a smarter brain. Dr. Norman Doidge of Canada has written a book named "The Brain That Changes Itself". Neuroplasticity is now accepted as true science. You should read his book.

You already have in essence two brains. One in the skull and one in the gut. There is enough volume of nerve cells in the gut to make up the volume of a second brain. They talk to one another via the vagus nerve.

One school of thought postulates that Parkinson's Disease starts in the gut, which sends retrograde nerve signals to the midbrain ganglia. Levodopa is produced in the substantia nigra. Abnormal levodopa metabolism governs the motor functions of the brain which characterize P.D. Electric probes directly in the brain can modify P.D. and MRI exposure of the brain can modify P.D.

A normal human brain weighs about three pounds. About 20% is proteins and the rest is mostly fat. At least 60% of the dry weight of the brain is lipids. Approximately 20% is cholesterol and most of the other 40% is DHA. Yes. You are a fathead.

The brain itself does not have pain receptors, so you cannot have pain in the brain.

INFRARED

The brain responds well to infrared energy.

Right now you can buy a vieLight Neuro Alpha unit for under $2000.00 to give yourself IR brain treatment. The unit has two parts. One covers the skull with clusters of units that emit IR waves that penetrate the skull bones and exposes the brain and vessels to IR.

The other part is an intra-nasal light that shines a 810 nano frequency signal that illuminates the base of the skull/brain. This completes the treatment of the brain from above and below. The nose to brain connection is the most direct pathway to the brain. Ask any cocaine sniffer.

AVAZZIA has protocols that treat from head to toe. It is the so-called "doc in a box". Avazzia Pro Sport units are the most expensive and versatile. They are self-contained portable frequency generators. Size is about that of mid-sized Remote TV controller. Battery Powered.

AVAZZIA PROSPORT is currently used by medical professionals including neurologists, orthopedists, chiropractors, dentists, sports medicine practitioners, acupuncturists and veterinarians.

Investigative work is continuing.

PROSPORT has many pre-programmed protocols, so you can start using the unit right out of the box. You just need some knowledge of the technology and it's possibilities. At least one hands-on class will be a big help.

DETA ELIS kills bacteria and viruses at their resonance frequency. All life-forms have a basic natural resonance frequency. Applying an external matching resonance frequency causes them to self-destruct.

SUMMARY

Everything cannot be included in a summary, but here goes: If you have been diagnosed with TYPE TWO DIABETES you can do a lot to manage your condition. Most important is to somehow regain insulin sensitivity. Nothing is as important as regaining insulin sensitivity. It cannot be emphasized too much that the key to overcoming diabetes is to regain sensitivity to insulin. Type 1 diabetics lack the ability to make any insulin.

You don't become type 2 diabetic from a lack of insulin. You become type 2 diabetic when you lose sensitivity to insulin. Goal is to restore sensitivity to low levels of insulin. You may need diabetes boot camp as a last resort.

A good place to start is with fasting. There are several regimens. Various degrees of mind resolution are needed to succeed at fasting.

My favorite is intermittent fasting with Bulletproof Coffee.

You would have begun the night before.

Stop eating three hours before bedtime.

Start with regular or decaf coffee.

Add MCT (preferably C8 Caprylic fraction) or organic grass-fed ghee.

Be sure to use a coffee-frother to emulsify the fat in MCT/ghee. Don't skip frothing.

Add some beef gelatin sourced from grass fed cows. This gets you a head start with protein.

DO NOT ADD MILK. It will deactivate polyphenols.

Take it black. Same for tea.

Add ribose sugar. It is less sweet than glucose and is needed for ATP as well as cardiac energy. If you still have a sweet-tooth add some stevia powder or liquid.

Take a green coffee chlorogenic pill together with bulletproof. Drink the bulletproof coffee with additives early in the day.

You will not be hungry till several hours later, maybe not even by noon (and beyond).

You would not have eaten since 8 PM the night before.

About sixteen hours of fasting would have passed.

Drink a protein smoothie. Try two boiled eggs with lots of grass fed butter.

Eat nutritious food. Avoid starches, carbohydrates and sugar.

If you are not a confirmed vegetarian, drink beef broth. Lots of it.

Eat a combination of proteins and fats.

Some proteins at each meal, but do not exceed 25 grams in any single meal.

You could drink bulletproof coffee again later in the day.

Cut out diet sodas entirely. Cut out corn syrup high fructose.

Drink good clean water. Try alkaline water made up with baking soda. The baking soda provides bicarbonate.

Follow with magnesium water made with carbonated water and magnesium carbonate powder. This supplies the magnesium. You need magnesium bicarbonate as the final product.

Be judicious in your meals. Try for organic vegetables if you can afford it.

Eat organic eggs too. Do not eat fats and carbohydrates together.

Increase Omega 3 intake.

Try to shift from:

Carbohydrates, starch, sugar, and insulin... regimen To fats, ketones, and lipase... regimen.

Dr. Mercola recommends that you get 70% to 80% of your calories from healthy fats. You need a big leap of faith for you wrap your head around that concept, but he builds a persuasive and logical case for his argument. His book : FAT FOR FUEL

Concentrate your eating into the window between noon (or later) and six or seven at night. Stop eating three hours before bedtime.

REPEAT CYCLE next day and succeeding days.

You need to add judicious minerals and vitamins and some sea salt. Current research shows that plastic residues are beginning to be found in sea salt, along with radioactive elements from Fukushima.

Be sure to take CoQ10, vitamin D, PQQ, pterostilbene, niacinamide, a probiotic, glutathione and whatever you decide in conjunction with your medical team. Add bicarbonates to balance your pH.

Include magnesium as a supplement. Insulin and magnesium need each other.

A BDNF (brain derived neurotropic factor) supplement will bring you right up to date.

Stay away from inflammatory foods. Sugar and Omega 6 fats are inflammatory.

The best known anti-inflammatory sources are Omega 3s and circumin in turmeric.

"Golden milk" is made with a combination of ground turmeric powder, ginger powder, galangal powder, cinnamon powder, crushed black-peppper and fat such as ghee to make the turmeric bio-available.

Turmeric for circumin is fat soluble. Add enough milk and heat.

Drink golden milk to reduce inflammation. It should reduce CRP and HOMOCYSTEINE. Both are markers of inflammation.

Electric medicine is in its infancy and the future is wide open. Keep an eye out for new developments.

I hope that you have benefited in some manner from this book and that you have been exposed to some new ideas or at least gained some new insights.

Be good to yourself.

THANKS FOR TAKING

THIS JOURNEY WITH ME.

READING LIST

The Body Electric   R.O. Becker & Gary Sheldon

ISBN 9780688 06971-1

The PEO Solution   Peskin & Rowen

ISBN 978 09882780 3-5

Radiant Health   Peskin with Marcus Conyers

ASIN B000XYMY0M

The Fat Switch   Richard J Johnson

ISBN 978 0 615 64800 2

Healing Fats   Alex Bradford

ISBN 978 0 6923866 4 4

Tripping Over The Truth   Travis Christofferson

ISBN 9781500600310

Healing Is Voltage   Jerry Tennant

ISBN 978 1453649169

PEMF   Bryant Meyers

ISBN 978 1452579221

There Is A Cure For Diabetes   Gabriel Cousens

ISBN 978 1 58394-544 5

The Resistant Starch Diet   Gregory Stevens

ASINB00O99UCJC

Current Medicine   John Hache & Lorraine Hache

ISBN 9781511870009

Head Strong   Dave Asprey

ISBN 9780062652416

Younger   Sara Gottfried

ISBN 9780062316271

Fat For Fuel   Joseph Mercola

ISBN 9781401953775

The End of Alzheimer's   Dale E. Brederson

ISBN 9780735216204

ABOUT THE AUTHOR

The author graduated from University of Southern California School of Medicine. Currently known as Keck-School of Medicine.-USC.

He served internship, residency and fellowship at the largest teaching hospital in the nation. He is board certified as a specialist in two separate disciplines by the American Board of Medical Specialties.

This gives him a good background for observing the practice of medicine. And for commenting on management of diabetes.

He has been diagnosed with diabetes for over twenty-five years, and has had first hand experience of how diabetes has been treated symptomatically over a long time.

He personally has escaped the potential bad effects of diabetic complications. He has normal renal functions. Normal neurologic examinations. No peripheral neuropathy. Normal opthalmologic examinations with no diabetic retinopathy. Normal small vessels in the lower extremities and feet. Normal digestive status. Normal gastrointestinal functions. Low risk for cardiac disease. Normal lipids. LDL profile predominantly large fluffy particles. Low HDL to triglyceride ratio.

He lives with his spouse of fifty-five years in Southern California.

DIABETES NUTRITION
and
ELECTRIC MEDICINE

The author graduated from University Of Southern California School of Medicine. He served internship, residency and fellowship at the largest teaching hospital in the nation. He is board certified as a specialist in two separate specialties by the American Board of Medical Specialties.

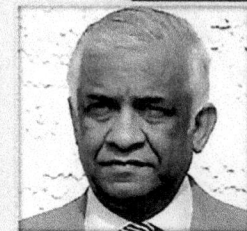

This gives him a good background for observing the practice of medicine. And for commenting on management of diabetes.

He has been diagnosed with diabetes for over twenty-five years, and has had first hand experience of how diabetes has been treated symptomatically over a long time.

He personally has escaped the potential bad effects of diabetic complications.
- He has normal renal functions.
- Normal neurologic examinations.
- No peripheral neuropathy _
- Normal opthalmologic examinations with no diabetic retinopathy.
- Normal small vessels in the lower extremities and feet. Normal digestive status.
- Normal gastrointestinal functions.
- Low risk for cardiac disease.
- Normal lipids.
- LDL profile predominantly large fluffy particles.
- Low HDL to triglyceride ratio.

He lives with his spouse of fifty-five years in southern California.

www.ingramcontent.com/pod-product-compliance
Lightning Source LLC
Chambersburg PA
CBHW051706170526
45167CB00002B/556